# A Little Pregnant

# A Little Pregnant

## Our Memoir of Fertility, Infertility, and a Marriage

Linda Carbone and Ed Decker

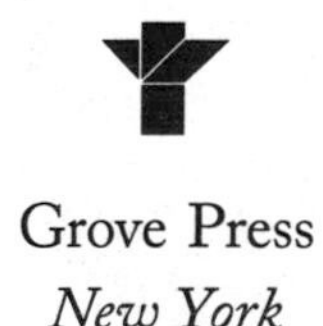

Grove Press
*New York*

*Published simultaneously in Canada*
*Printed in the United States of America*

FIRST PAPERBACK EDITION

Library of Congress Cataloging-in-Publication Data

Carbone, Linda.
A little pregnant : our memoir of fertility, infertility, and a marriage / Linda Carbone and Ed Decker.
p. cm.
ISBN 0-8021-3745-8 (pbk.)
1. Carbone, Linda. 2. Infertility, Female—Patients—Biography. 3. Decker, Ed. 4. Human reproductive technology. I. Decker, Ed. II. Title.
RG201.C28 1999
362.1'98178'0092—dc21
[B] 99-19217
CIP

Design by Laura Hammond Hough

Grove Press
841 Broadway
New York, NY 10003

01 02 03 04 10 9 8 7 6 5 4 3 2 1

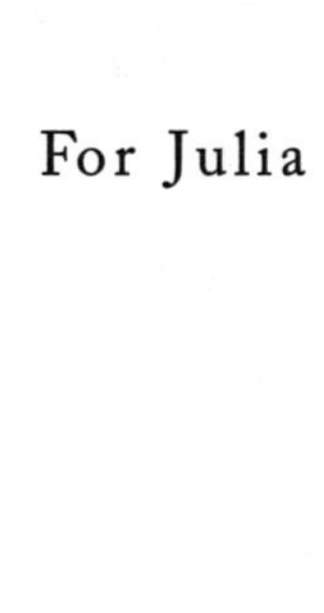

For Julia

Were it possible for us to see further than our knowledge reaches, and yet a little way beyond the outworks of our divining, perhaps we would endure our sadnesses with greater confidence than our joys. For they are the moments when something new has entered into us, something unknown; our feelings grow mute in shy perplexity, everything in us withdraws, a stillness comes, and the new, which no one knows, stands in the midst of it and is silent.

—Rilke, *Letters to a Young Poet*

# Chapter 1
# Date of Confinement

"You were born in a snowstorm," it would have begun. "It snowed so hard the day you were born, we didn't think we'd make it to the hospital on time." The first personal legend for my son or daughter, who would have taken it in with a shy smile at first, in later years nodding, knowing the details by heart.

They had shown me the due date on a cardboard wheel in the obstetrician's office. The energies of the cosmos and the zodiac had swirled together with my body to determine this fine point in time. "E.D.C.," they called it there, for Expected Date of Confinement—an archaic, faintly misogynistic term no one had ever bothered to change. Mine would be January 12.

I suppose I should have covered my eyes and ears, knowing the history of my previous conceptions, hard-won and hard-lost. But against my nature, perhaps against Nature itself, I felt optimistic. A pathetic optimism, the kind a pessimist occasionally gets. For I am not the silver-lining type. And I had allowed myself to be pinned in place by thousands of tiny nails, a consenting Gulliver, immobilized by the medical and psychological restraints imposed by infertility.

There had been others, two others—the first fruits, offered to appease the gods—but this was the last, best hope, made real by a cardboard pinwheel that gave me the hard nugget of a month and a day to hold on to. I had seen the embryonic outline this time on a sonogram, the one that was supposed to confirm the positive blood test by showing its little heartbeat.

I had been so sure this time that I almost didn't bother going for the verification. Peppermints had suddenly begun to nauseate me, and my nipples had turned to rubber. "There aren't that many highs in life," Karen, the coordinator at the fertility clinic, had said. "Go and see the heartbeat."

The dark image I saw had the hunch and curve I recognized from pictures. But it had no heart to beat. To make sure, the technician kept enlarging it until the screen was filled with its motionless hulk. Its shape, the kindly doctor told me after I got dressed, gave a clue to its trouble. It showed signs, he explained, that it might be about to "crumple"—an unmistakable word, with its unforgiving "k" sound and the abrupt energy of that "p."

Of the millions of words I have heard, thought, and spoken about infertility in the seven years my husband and I tried to make a baby, it's the word "crumple" that sticks with me this January 12, as I roam unconfined on my Date of Confinement. In New York's record-breaking snowfall in the winter of 1994, it is the legacy of my infertility that I carry with me, not my baby.

Infertility is what I do. It's my vocation: I don't get pregnant, or I don't stay pregnant. I'm good at it. I've been more successful at it than at anything else I've tried as an adult. My infertility is a layered, soft thing, spun of gossamer and tears. It will disintegrate if I touch it. So I give it substance in other ways.

I have a record of every date on which I menstruated and ovulated during the last seven years. Also every date my husband and I had intercourse. I could draw charts and graphs—"Here's where I didn't get pregnant *that* month"—to illustrate our childlessness. The ritual and science of failure.

When Ed and I started out, it seemed clear that determination and the right medical care would get us there. But we had to live in the world until then. And on the bad days, everyone I saw, even the men, seemed to be effortlessly, abundantly pregnant. How dare they?

But it wasn't just pregnant people and babies—babies in blankets, babies in strollers, babies cooing, babies shrieking, everywhere babies, babies, babies—who had the power to stun. Every human being I saw was a reminder that I could not make one of those. It seemed mythical, a compelling fiction, that we had all started out from the successful union of egg and sperm successfully housed in a successful uterus.

I wasn't sick, but over the years I collected the names of diseases and conditions that applied to me. I wasn't dying, but I could not give life. I claimed a new terrain between the ill and the well, and there I alternated between hope and cynicism daily, monthly, yearly: we could be helped/we would never be parents; we had diseases that could be treated/we were losing incalculable, irretrievable time and money on a doomed quest.

As the diagnoses and treatments accumulated, I gradually built up a vocabulary of loss: endometriosis, varicocele, curettage, fetal demise. If worst came to worst, there was the terrible miracle of reproductive technology. And it works, sort of. It made me a little pregnant.

But first, I had to prepare myself. I had to become somebody else. Somebody capable of undergoing surgery after surgery, submitting to six months of medically induced menopause at age thirty-two, laying hot compresses of boiled ginger root across her midsection, chanting novenas in secular spots.

Ed and I traveled to California to continue treatment when the doctor we liked moved there. We traveled to Queens to call on the services of an acupuncturist. I rekindled a childhood pen pal correspondence in France in order to take advantage of the much cheaper fertility drugs in that country.

My break with the Catholic Church in junior high didn't stop me from collecting the little laminated cards my sister gave me with incantations to the Virgin Mary and St. Gerard for motherhood. And toward the end, I began a series of experimental blood transfusions without realizing that they would have run into tens of thousands of dollars.

We tried everything: the sacred and the profane, the medical and the marginal, the cutting edge and the fringe. No gesture seemed too far-fetched. The more extreme, we thought, the more likely it would be to form another piece of the humorous, heartbreaking story we would tell once our parenthood was secured. We got the humor and the heartbreak, anyway.

There was the doctor who forgot to tell me that the diagnostic procedure he would be performing on me would put me in the long lineup of that morning's abortions. There was the radiologist whose job it was to report my uterine X rays to my doctor, but who couldn't keep his unfounded suspicions of endometrial cancer to himself. There were the slapstick maneuvers involved in getting the adjustable in vitro table to hoist my large frame (I'm nearly 5'10") into the appropriate angle for the transfer of precious embryos.

And then there was Dr. Gold, my friend and confidant through the long, confusing years. From the start, he took a special interest in my case. I basked in his quirky attentiveness. I liked his directness, his Jewishness, his delicate surgeon's hands, his birdlike movements. With his close-cropped black hair, wire-rim glasses, and scaled-down facial features, he was endearing, irresistible: Albert Brooks in surgical scrubs. For better or worse, I couldn't have stuck it out without his intimate involvement.

I gave myself over to my infertility as to an inevitable trial, a test of will, of faith, of reason. Each monthly cycle, each new treatment, seemed the small, logical next step in a reasonable sequence. In the medical miasma, I couldn't see the incremental madness. I saw only myself, trying to be a good patient, addled but agreeable; my husband, with his unexpected, intense love that both anchored and buoyed me, whose longing for fatherhood was so genuine that I ached to be able to offer it to him; and my doctor—energetic, compassionate, and personally rooting for me. The barren woman's ménage à trois.

But even as Ed and I dutifully turned to successively more complicated treatments, as to the stations of some powerful pagan's cross, I had a gnawing feeling that some unnameable sequence of wrong choices and the earth's damaged environment itself had already preordained our childlessness. We were canaries in the coal mine, hallucinating in our asphyxiation that our rescuers were only shovelfuls away.

And early on, I knew that I didn't necessarily want a child—no more than I wanted everything I had ever longed for and didn't have. Like a peaceful childhood with the kind of father who would have taught me to dance by lifting me on top of his shoes and waltzing me around the room. Or getting back my best friend, Kathy, whose life ended at twenty-four in the fiery crash of a small plane in Vermont.

The difference here was that I could place responsibility for having a baby in the hands of medical authorities. They were our collaborators, our dream-catchers, dangling before us the constant promise of possible parenthood, a promise they had been known to keep. I threw myself at them as though they could give me everything I had ever wanted—as though, if only I could have this, I would never want anything again.

I think I also embraced my infertility for its drama and pathos. I love movies that make me cry, music in minor chords, books that let sorrow wash over me. Even in real life, sadness often feels more real to me than the alternatives. It touches a depth nothing else can reach. As my infertility gained ascendancy, it exploited that feeling in me. "You want sad?" it jeered. "I'll give you sad."

Even worse, it threatened to turn me wholly inward, shrinking my perspective down to the size of my uterus. On the day I found out that our attempt at in vitro fertilization had failed, in 1992, I saw the first photographs of the wasted bodies of Somali children on the front page of the *New York Times.* Who in God's name did I think I was?

Someday, I thought, I might try to make sense of the ordeal by writing about it. Would that give me perspective? If I couldn't be pregnant, maybe at least I could be poignant.

Now that my seven years' bad luck have ended—my penance for mirrors and commandments I don't remember breaking—and now that I can tally up the number of surgeries and miscarriages, reckon what has been lost and what gained, along with the sorrow and the relief, I also feel surprise that I took it that far. Part of me feels that I've been had, humiliated, given a metaphysical wedgie. Trying to have a child turned out to be no different from trying to be Bolivian or trying to have small feet.

But I was mesmerized by the process, so that as I progressed through each complex, futile stage, I was vaguely aware of having the choice of either jolting myself awake or just working it into the dream, the fever dream it took me seven years to wake up from. Now, sweating and disoriented, the frown of troubled sleep still upon me and the blood still roiling in my ears, I search frantically for some familiar sign of who I was back before the fever took hold.

## Chapter 2

# Discard Artichokes Before Reaching Orgasm

I'm scanning the signs above the aisles in the Grand Union on Eighty-sixth Street. I steer no cart, swing no basket, because I'm here to purchase only one item. Something that will help determine whether I can father a child: a jar of artichokes.

No, I didn't read about a longitudinal study of Harvard University graduates revealing that artichoke consumption improves sperm count. I seek the jar itself because, properly sterilized, it will make a practical container for transporting my semen to the clinic that will analyze it tomorrow morning.

This is hardly the scenario I anticipated when Linda and I began trying to conceive in August 1986, sixteen months ago. By now there should be a tiny baby in our apartment, suckling at Linda's breast and being rocked back and forth in her maternal lap. Instead, Linda sits at home reading the newspaper rather than Dr. Spock, her stomach flat from months of abdominal conditioning with a Jane Fonda fitness video and showing no signs of expanding.

Our timing for starting a family had seemed perfect that summer. We were both in good health. My career as a copywriter at an ad agency was secure, Linda's as a freelance editor was steady. Linda had just returned from a month in London, not as a tourist but as a literature student at the University of London. And me? I had just climbed a mountain. While Linda was across the Atlantic I had driven deep into Maine, alone, then spent nine hours clawing my way to the top of Mount Katahdin and down again, elevation a mile-plus. My knees were shot for a month afterward, but I had done it. It was a memory under lock and key, no longer a goal that might become more elusive after parenthood redefined my life.

And there was love, too. I had had the good judgment—or good luck—to marry someone who was my best friend as well as my lover, something a number of my divorced friends had failed to do. Linda and I were soulmates who never tired of each other's company, who gladly spent hours talking about everything or nothing. We had become insightful commentators on the dynamics of our families, and remained eager to learn more about each other as our years together added up. And by 1986, seven years after our first date for lunch at a Manhattan tavern, I was certain we had closed any communication gaps and flushed out any secrets about ourselves that over time could have festered into serious differences. Our marriage had fused us into a single entity with no seams or fault lines, a bond that would surely remain intact through the rigors and uncertainties of parenthood.

I thought I'd make a good father, maybe even a great one. Ever since kids began appearing in the families of relatives and friends, I'd gotten a tremendous kick out of playing with them. Often I was the only large person willing to trade in my adult credentials to spend the evening in a child's world. It was irresistible to me. Where else could I become an instant superman, using my superstrength to toss toddlers skyward and my supernatural powers to make a croquet ball and a Q-Tip swab fall to the ground at equal speed?

Of course, I realized that there was a lot more to being a father than juggling tennis balls and making monkey faces. But I was pretty sure I could handle the serious stuff, too. I'd taught preschoolers who were petrified of the water how to swim when I was a lifeguard in college. I'd been a Big Brother who helped an emotionally disturbed boy overcome his fear of baseball, roller skating, and life. I had even roamed through the neighborhood and handed out goodies to the local trick-or-treaters one Halloween, in case they never made it to my apartment. So what if some kid in a ghost costume reported me to his mother and two police cars screeched to a halt around me as I walked up to my front door? Sure, I had what it took to be a good Dad.

I supposed that a large part of my reason for wanting to be a father was to revisit my own childhood. It seemed like I was the only person I knew whose early years weren't tainted by some shadow of unpleasantness—an uncaring father, an overbearing mother, or some inescapable tragedy. I'd grown up in a house with hardworking and caring parents, a fun sister, a wise grandmother. There were no dark periods, just occasional lamenting about not having a girlfriend or not being a star on some athletic team.

Watching the immense pleasure my sister, Chris, took in her children had also made it clear that having kids was a special privilege. I also thought that she was a wonderful mother in every sense, and that I was learning invaluable parenting skills by watching her in action.

I'd never even questioned my desire to have kids. To me, parenthood was one of the ultimate experiences of life, on equal footing with falling in love and finding a vocation. Linda, on the other hand, had early on told me she had mixed feelings about parenthood, and these feelings didn't change after we got married in 1982. She didn't detect any maternal instinct stirring when she saw other mothers with their progeny, was fairly certain she could lead a fully satisfying life without children, and wasn't sure if she could make the necessary sacrifices or commitment involved in child-rearing. But she was only in her mid-twenties then; I figured that over time the instinct would kick in, or that a clearer vision of her mortality would convince her to add a branch to the family tree.

I tried to sway Linda by telling her how rewarding it would be to have a child, how it would bring a bounty of new happiness and fulfillment into our lives. How we would marvel at watching someone who was a part of us learn to walk, to talk, to read. How we'd share every step of this incredible being's development from cuddly armful to self-sufficient adult. She acknowledged all of these things as great moments, but wasn't sure she could embrace the whole package of motherhood. Eventually my response to Linda's "What if I don't change my mind about kids?" came down to this: nothing. I changed the subject or faded into silence, hoping to create a black hole that would suck her relationship-threatening words into a place from where they couldn't be pulled out again.

Not have kids? The notion was unthinkable to me. When I imagined a future without them, I saw Linda and me going to the movies and reading, friendless because everyone we knew was involved with their progeny, the hands on the clock whizzing around as our hair turned gray and our joints went stiff and our favorite movie stars died and the pages became brittle in our hands. I saw us sitting with polite smiles at gatherings on holidays and birthdays as we listened to stories of first words, first steps, first days at school, first boyfriends and girlfriends. "Nothing new with us" would be our rebuttal, year after year after year.

Linda also feared that having children might put us on a path toward stereotypical gender roles. She had kept her last name after marriage, and we'd always split our costs fifty-fifty. We even kept separate bank accounts. And after she moved into my apartment, she liked that we were together without resorting to the convention of marriage, that being crazy in love was all we needed to stay a couple.

I was pretty much in agreement with Linda on these matters, but after a year and a half of living together I became itchy to make it legal. By then I was approaching twenty-nine, and I felt compelled to get married before I turned thirty—as if unless I did, all the other milestones of my life, whatever they might be, would be a little late from then on. I also felt uncomfortable that my parents knew we were doing it without our having said "I do." I knew this seemed almost prudish by the standards of my generation, but I couldn't shake my concerns over their possible disapproval.

"Okay, but not yet," Linda said at our favorite restaurant one fall evening in 1981. I had just proposed to her after plopping down a vase with a single red rose, which I had been hiding inside my overcoat.

"We're going to stay together forever anyway," I countered. "Why not just make it official?"

Linda finally came around to marriage, in large part due to my intensive lobbying, and eventually to kids, too. The key impetus for Linda's shift on kids: her vivacious, beautiful niece, Andrea. Linda developed a special bond with Andrea that showed her the flip side of labor-intensive child-rearing. It brought a new kind of love into her life that helped her recognize the potential joys of motherhood.

Soon after our first forays into unprotected sex, a new life began taking shape in my crystal ball. I saw myself reading about Goldilocks, complete with gruff imitations of bear talk, with a little girl on my lap. Proudly listening to a little boy's thirtieth consecutive playing of "Chopsticks" on the piano. Throwing slow bounce passes to two little someones on a basketball court. I was reinventing myself, ready to discard my current identity for one that I coveted more than any other.

After six months of trying to make a baby, Linda told me her period was late. She wanted to take a pregnancy test right away. Overcome by superstition, I wanted to wait a few days. I felt it was presumptuous to confirm our pregnancy yet. Presumptuous in whose eyes? God's? The American Academy of Pediatrics'? I couldn't explain it, couldn't justify it by any rational means. I had tapped into a feeling from childhood, back when I feared finding my Christmas presents before they were wrapped and under the tree, as if I'd be punished by knowing too much too soon.

So we held off, against Linda's wishes, as she remained gift-wrapped for a full week. At work I stared at my computer monitor, visions of individual cells splitting into two, then four, then eight replacing the headlines and promotional blurbs I was editing. I saw mounds of Play-Doh morphing into cherubic faces, robotlike bodies constructing themselves out of Lego pieces. Then at night I'd lie in bed in the dark, allowing myself to smile just a little as I visualized a rich new life for myself as a father.

My pace slows as I turn left into the aisle with the canned vegetables. Finally I spot the distinctive jar, standing at attention amid the roasted peppers and pimientos. There are three brands, all of them in squat, wide containers. The design of the artichoke jar is ideal for capturing semen, the gaping mouth reducing a man's chances of missing the target and the thick glass unlikely to shatter if the jar should slip out of his hand and fall to the floor.

I reach for the jar and then stop—the artichokes sitting in olive oil look more like muscle tissue than vegetables. They remind me of the bottles of chicken embryos preserved in formaldehyde that were lined up on a table under the window in my eighth-grade science class. For ten months I was flanked by those unborn animals that were forever frozen at different stages of gestation. They mocked both life and death resting there, floating in liquid just as they had been when a future existence still beckoned.

Six days after Linda's missed period, on a Friday night, we were looking over dinner menus in a restaurant near my midtown office. I noticed that Linda was being very quiet and avoiding eye contact with me.

"I'm spotting," she said.

A chill vibrated my spine. Spotting. Drops of blood. It sounded so sinister, as if someone had just shot Linda under the table.

I paused a second or two, then stammered, "Is it still happening now?"

"Yeah."

"A lot? What does it mean?"

"Not a lot. It doesn't necessarily mean anything."

"But what could be causing it?"

"It happens to some women during pregnancy."

"How many?"

Linda looked down.

"Sorry," I said. "What should we do?"

"See if it stops."

I looked around the restaurant. Somebody from work was at a table across the room, but Linda's news made me feel like a stranger in my own life. I turned my head so the person wouldn't know I'd seen her.

The next morning I poured Linda's urine into the little reservoirs whose color changes would tell us yes or no. But we never got to see those changes; I accidentally knocked the vials into the sink. Afterward I felt stupid but also relieved, as if my mistake had actually destroyed bad news.

After dinner that night Linda took to her bed, alternating between sleep and severe cramps. I wanted so much to reach out to her, to deflect some of her pain or absorb it into myself, but there was nothing I could do. I sensed that she didn't want me there, that I was a distraction from her efforts to will away her agony. For much of the evening I sat numbly in the living room watching *West Side Story* on television, feeling a tremor every time I heard her whimper behind the living room wall. Linda ended up sitting hunched over in the empty bathtub, shivering. I sat on the edge, but she pushed my hand away. Maybe it was just the reflex of someone in pain; I never asked her.

The scene was eerily familiar. A year before, a food processor blade had fallen out of a kitchen cabinet and buzz-sawed into Linda's big toe, the blood spurting out in a waterfall. I quickly determined that there was no time to dial 911, then took her into the bathroom, hoisted her foot over the bathtub, and held the sides of the wound together for an hour and a half to stop the flow. I remained completely calm as Linda wavered on the verge of vomiting and fainting with her head over the sink. I wasn't the least bit squeamish as I leaned over the blood-spattered tub and my blood-soaked hands. My senses took in nothing but the essentials: my hands, her toe. After the bleeding stopped I guided Linda to the bed, then took her sliced leather flip-flop down the hall and threw it in the garbage chute. On the way back, my knees buckled and I collapsed against the wall of the hallway, shaking uncontrollably. I waited until I was stable again, then went back into the apartment. A rush of pride swept through me as I looked at Linda, safe and sleeping on the bed. I had never been tested like this before, and I had passed.

In a way, Linda's life-threatening night had taxed my nerves less than her miscarriage had, probably because I could do something to combat her wound. After the miscarriage I could do nothing except hover over her until she fell asleep. The next morning I awoke before her. I touched her gently on her thigh with one finger, hoping that I could conduct away whatever pain she would otherwise feel when she awoke. I wanted to guard her somehow against both physical distress and the shock of remembering what had happened the day before.

What I failed to anticipate was the fallout that landed on me when we tried to conceive again the next month. My body sabotaged our efforts within seconds after intercourse began, my penis going numb and limp like an animal speared by an anesthetizing dart. Despite our best erotic efforts, nothing seemed to help. I had not been aware of the slightest tension beforehand; it was as if a third party had turned a spigot cutting off the blood supply.

Two days later it happened again, then again two days after that, passing us through peak ovulation with not a single sperm emerging from my body. Linda was very sympathetic, telling me not to worry, next month would be fine. I wasn't so sure. What if some new physical problem had wormed its way into me? Or what if a mental block had been lodged in my head, my subconscious mind's way to protect Linda against any more doomed pregnancies?

I would never know for sure what caused my problem. The next month it was gone, without my having consulted a shrink, urologist, or hypnotist. My demon had been exorcised as mysteriously as it had invaded me. But while I retained my potency as the year proceeded, our attempts at conception became more and more like training sessions. Linda's monthly release of blood was no longer proof that she could have a baby, but a demonstration of life not granted.

Meanwhile the population boomed around us. A good friend from college had a baby boy. My cousin in Maine sired a baby girl. I could feel the ceiling of my happiness lowering above me, as these new tiny creatures accumulated below. It was no longer easy for me to entertain the little ones who had always been my biggest fans. I still gravitated toward the kids at social gatherings, but now it seemed more like an obligation than an opportunity for fun.

On one slow day at the agency, I attempted to stave off depression by writing down a list of people who don't have children. Priests. Hermaphrodites. James Bond. Winnie the Pooh. As the list became more and more absurd, a hint of a smile tempered my gloom.

Slight paranoia stalks me as I head toward the "10 Items or Less" express cashier with my artichokes. My fellow shoppers are looking at my little jar, then at me, with disdain, I'm sure of it. Thought balloons pop out of their heads. "I know what you're going to do with that thing, you perve," thinks a woman by produce. "Couldn't you at least get one of those blowup dolls on Forty-second Street?" questions an elderly man picking over some fruit. "Wait, everybody," pleads my own balloon. "This act of autoeroticism is fully sanctioned by the medical community. It's not like I *want* to have an orgasm!"

As I revolve the artichoke jar around in my hand, I keep telling myself that this test is only a formality. A man's fertility is easier to confirm than a woman's, so it makes sense for me to get checked out first. But I'm afraid that opening the jar will uncover dreaded truths I have been hiding from for years. Like the time in college when I had an allergic reaction to a sulfa drug that left my pud shriveled and made the blood rush to my hands. Or, worse, an episode when I was a teenager that has haunted me, but that I've thought too bizarre or even perverse to mention to anyone.

I was fourteen, and my friend Tom and I were seeing how long we could hold a pull-up position on a chinning bar mounted in a doorway of my house. We were always creating new types of sporting events, and this was part of an indoor pentathlon competition I had devised for after-school diversion in the long, cold months before baseball season started.

After Tom maxed out at one minute and forty seconds, I assumed there was no way I could beat him. The guy had already whipped me in the upstairs/downstairs race, water-drinking endurance event, bread-swallowing sprint, and Fig Newtons–eating marathon.

To improve my motivation in the final event, I pretended to be hanging over a hundred-foot gorge as my sweaty hands locked on to the cool metal tubing. The tactic worked; soon I had passed the ninety-second mark. My arms were shaking like they were clutching a jackhammer, but I forced myself to concentrate; there was no way I'd allow Tom to win every event on my home turf.

At the two-minute mark, the intense pain in my shoulders shifted into the background and I felt what seemed like a slight electric current rippling through my groin. At first this made me queasy; then it was faintly pleasurable. After sensing a rush of heat into my pud, I collapsed to the floor. My time: two minutes, fourteen seconds.

After Tom went home, I hurried to the bathroom to investigate and found the horrifying evidence: a dollop of semen looking like a dead worm hanging out of my dick. I stumbled backward at the sight, as if trying to move away from my own body. It was the first time I'd seen the substance out of the context of a wet dream. Somehow I had crossed the barrier between pain and pleasure, and my body had launched a counter-attack of ecstasy against the stress of my exertion.

I'd almost forgotten about this episode over the years. But now, as my reproductive machinery is about to come under close scrutiny, I'm wondering if my victory in that long-ago suspension over cheap linoleum could have cost me my chance at fatherhood.

I spill the artichokes directly into the garbage in my kitchen, their edibility compromised by the fate of their container. It reminds me of a scene from *Portnoy's Complaint* in which the protagonist jerks off into a piece of meat that his mother then cooks for dinner.

It takes Linda ten minutes to wash all the dinner dishes. It takes me fifteen to wash out my one jar. Squirting the dish-washing liquid into its gaping maw reminds me that I'll be aiming my own fluid at the same spot tomorrow. I want to smash the glass, take Linda in the bedroom, and have wild sex in some new position that would produce not one, but two healthy embryos.

Soon the images vanish, evaporating with the steam rising from the pot of boiling water that I now put the jar in for thirty minutes of sterilization, the word "sterilization" echoing ominously in my head. I will not take any shortcuts here; for all I know, one shred of vegetable matter or one microdrop of olive oil could wipe out a hundred million sperm. I'm back in high school chemistry, washing out flasks before weighing tiny amounts of powder on Mettler balances calibrated in milligrams.

I awake early the next morning, well before Linda's alarm clock sounds. She's offered her companionship for the occasion, but I decline; I need total control over the ejaculation to make sure I don't miss the jar. As I walk toward the living room, I feel as if I'm about to have an affair, with my wife twenty feet away.

On the kitchen counter sits my accomplice in this one-morning stand. Next to it is a roll of masking tape; I'll be using a strip of it to label my jar. I wonder what I'll write. "Ed's Sperm"? "Semen by Decker"?

Then a jolt of anxiety courses through me—what if I panic and can't get an erection? I should have rented an X-rated video. Now I have to rely entirely on my own imagination. What if the cat comes in and starts rubbing against me? Things could get very sordid.

I manage to dredge up a scene from a porn movie I saw as a teenager—a woman in a bathroom with a plumber who does a lot more than unclog her shower drain—and make it to the finish line. The jar feels cold against my dick, but my aim remains true.

Relief joins the usual feeling of serenity as I carefully tighten the lid onto the artichoke jar. I shower and get dressed quickly, wrapping my cargo in a sock and holding it inside my coat against the November chill as I leave the building. Just my luck that I have to do this on a frigid day. My sperm will probably perish like Napoleon's soldiers in the Russian winter.

On the subway ride to the lab, I picture the jar slipping out of my hands and onto the tracks. An infertile man mugging me for my sperm. Opening my coat at the lab to reveal a jar still filled with artichokes. Somehow I make it safely through six subway stops, then elevate to ground level without releasing my death grip on the hidden jar. I scan the area to make sure no one I know is outside the clinic, then walk inside. I place my jar in its plastic bag on the desk, telling the receptionist that I'm leaving a sample. "A sample of *what*?" I imagine her saying. "Oh my God, what is that, *cum*?" All she says is, "Thank you. You're all set."

I feel a sense of freedom going outside, as if I can play hooky from work today, go out for a big breakfast, see a movie. It's like heading out of school after the last final exam.

Then I become Fred MacMurray walking down the street in *Double Indemnity* after he's murdered someone, when he starts to become edgy because he can't hear his own footsteps. *The walk of a dead man,* he says. Now that I've handed off that sample, my manhood is under investigation. Maybe my dream of being a father will only ever be a dream. My mouth, watering minutes ago for a Spanish omelet, goes dry. With every step I become more convinced that they'll find something very bad in that artichoke jar.

But they don't. "Your test was completely normal; good count and movement," a woman tells me when I call the lab from work two days later. She might as well be Linda telling me she's pregnant again. I almost throw the receiver into the air in exultation at my acquittal.

"It's normal. Totally, absolutely normal," I tell Linda excitedly when I call her, seconds after hearing the news myself. "Good, hon," she says. Silence. Then my stupidly belated recognition: if I'm okay, Linda isn't.

# Chapter 3

# Baby Steps

I'm not sure when it began. It might have been the summer after I turned ten, when I got my first period. Or sometime during college when I learned, as all young women do, to trespass my own physical boundaries and impose or impale myself onto foreign objects: contact lenses, Tampax, penises. Or it might have been later in my twenties, when I looked at a young girl on the crosstown bus and thought, for the first time, not of the young me but of the possibility of a daughter.

At some moment between each of these revelations and the afternoon I found myself outside a gynecologist's office on the Upper East Side clutching a medical reimbursement slip with the word "infertility" neatly filled in, I became a woman who could not be a mother. I strapped myself tightly to the doctors, the treatments, the terminology, the whole warped merry-go-round that would carry me through my thirties in the harrowing and exhilarating attempts to coax my earnest but incompetent reproductive system into performing the dazzling, prosaic feat for which it was intended.

But the beginning, the real beginning, is hard to pin down. One beginning was that of Ed and me as a couple. We met at work, in the midtown Manhattan offices of an educational book publisher, me one year out of college, Ed three years older and on his second job. He was slowly, vaguely coming out of a two-year courtship. I was . . . well, let's just say that I had a hard time being myself around men. In high school I wondered where the other girls had learned to flirt, how they could go from talking about a boy they liked to holding hands with him. There was the oddball pseudo-romance here and there, and the steadfast true love of my adolescence, George Harrison. (A healthy improvement over my first crush: Moe.) I went through the obligatory steps of growing up in America—losing my virginity, losing my religion—but I didn't learn how to relax around guys until I fell in love with one and got married. And then they were suddenly off-limits.

I did not have the kind of physique that boys dreamed of. Oh, I developed early, all right. I was wearing my first brassiere in the fourth grade, camouflaging it under a scoop-necked undershirt for fear that its straps would give me away through my clothes. I think the boys in my class were too little even to joke about it or pretend to want me—I was more like their mother than their dream girl. Add to that my pathological shyness and grape-stomper's hips and legs, and it was clear there was little to advance my social development as a young girl in a working-class Long Island suburb.

I'm tall, and I got tall fast. As young as nine or ten, I'd get mistaken for a teacher from the back in school hallways. Worse, I was a straight-A student, I wore glasses from fifth grade until my second year of college, and I went through my entire adolescence being told by strangers to smile. Did everyone, I wondered, march around their junior high halls with a Cheshire grin plastered across their faces? What was it about my neutral expression that made people think I was sad?

In high school and again in college, I'd carried a torch for a tall, blond athlete I barely spoke to. When I took my first job, as an editorial assistant with a textbook publisher, I fell for another tall, blond athlete. Once Ed and I spoke—when our bosses became involved in a joint project—we dated feverishly, intensely, a young couple in New York City dazzled by each other and by the impossibly romantic backdrop to their young love. It was grand love on a grand scale, although we were broke. Ed was the first guy I'd met who didn't get thrown into an erotic tailspin when he met my roommate, a good friend from college who was thin and beautiful and knew how to wield her arms and her hair to sexy effect. When I asked him what he thought of her, he said, "Now, which one is that again?" Okay, now I was in love.

Shy as we both were, we couldn't stop talking. And we couldn't stand being apart. He was so tall that my head bent back at a sharp angle to my body when we kissed. I knew inside of a few weeks that we'd be together for keeps. Inside of a few months, we were living together, and two years later we'd become one of the thousands of young married couples in New York.

But this young couple is so in love, feels so protected by their love, that they are somehow undeterred by an undiscussed difference they are aware of going into the marriage. The husband is positive he wants children; the wife appears to have no real opinion on the subject but, if pressed, will say she simply can't picture a life with kids, has never really thought much about it. This would be enough to keep many a couple from heading down the aisle, but how do we handle it? We don't. We don't even talk about it, except to establish that Ed feels certain I will come around, feels he knows me well enough to take the chance. Me? I'm head over heels with a tall, blond athlete who loves me back. I'm not looking any further than that at the moment.

When I was growing up, in the sixties and seventies, having kids just wasn't a topic among my friends and me. We all had ethnic last names and we all had top grades. Many of us also had trouble at home, and we were thinking more about how not to repeat the pattern than about how to perpetuate it. Our fathers were tradesmen (laying bricks, installing floors) or, like my father, civil servants (he worked for the post office in the next town). Lots of them worked at the defense plants whose names—Grumman, Republic, Fairchild, Sperry—studded our consciousness, where the veterans of one war made weapons for another war.

The problem was that there was no defense against these gruff men once they came home at night, perpetually hot under the blue collar. There was no physical violence in my circle, only a different kind of treachery: either neglect or the constant growl of rage—insatiable, irrational rage, the men holding court in the evening as they couldn't during the day, teaching their daughters all about fear and indifference without also teaching us about fairness or compassion or self-respect. These we would gather slowly, as we could, over many years, coming to them fresh in our twenties and thirties after the freeing shock of college and the heartrending kindness of other people's affection.

Those of our mothers who worked took jobs at Sears or as secretaries with small local companies. It was always referred to as "helping out." My mother, a talented seamstress who'd designed and made coats, slipcovers, and wedding gowns, helped out at a state psychiatric hospital, sewing the hems onto sheets and pillowcases. A war bride from England (well, two years after the war, without much romance or speed), she valued productivity, thrift, and the ability to withstand hardship.

She'd gone to work at fourteen in London the year World War II got under way, and lived out her teenage years amid its terrors and deprivations. Most of our fathers had fought in the war, but I had the only mother who'd seen it. She was full of stories we found dramatic and exciting from our safe remove, but only with the most insistent prodding could we get her to retell the one about stepping out for a pack of cigarettes while many of her coworkers at the sewing factory got injured or killed by flying glass caused by a bombing. (The image of her girlfriend staggering across the room with an enormous piece of jagged glass in her chest before collapsing into death is with me still. And of other women found later in the branches of nearby trees.) Or the one about running home from the train station late one night, dodging huge pieces of shrapnel that fell all around her like rain. After leaving England, I don't think the feeling ever quite left her that she was lucky just to be out of the war zone.

She kept our house immaculately clean and kept as busy as she could within it. She loved her American children with a desperate, fearful love, born of unentitlement, self-effacement, and the refusal to forgive herself for having left her family back in England. We felt a saintly devotion and love toward her, but it never seemed quite enough.

My two older sisters and I were wary partners, listening to our radios and watching television while our childhoods passed us by, learning to stay invisible so as not to set anything off. I got through by making sure the worlds of home and school did not touch. It wasn't until talking to Ed about it that I realized I remembered almost nothing before the age of about ten except the smell of new cloth on the first day of school; every year my mother would have us flip through the Butterick and Simplicity pattern books the big department stores had on podiums in those days and then let us choose fabric for two new dresses. To me, childhood was a strange period to be jumped past so that you could get to the next stage, where everything would begin.

But three blissful years into our marriage, the topic of our own children began to be raised. I usually winced and tried to put off discussing it, but by four years into the marriage there was no getting around it. As far as Ed was concerned, it was time. The notion of parenthood not only felt foreign to me, but I was afraid there'd be no space or breath again—not because someone in the house would be breathing fire, but because I'd seen parents who had nothing left over once they'd taken care of their kids. I couldn't imagine being able to summon the manic energy or the utter self-sacrifice that children seemed to require and still cling to a semblance of my own grown-up life.

But Ed's firm desire for children held up against my wobbly uncertainty, felt but inexpressible then. I squeezed in some graduate school and a summer study trip to Europe without him, then declared myself ready. I didn't so much give it thought—I didn't know how to—as prepare to cash in a voucher I'd been carrying around in my back pocket for a long time.

We started somewhere, in some agreed-upon month after I turned thirty, but the first obstruction is a lot clearer in my mind. By this time I'd become a freelance editor and Ed was working for an ad agency. Six or so months after I packed up my diaphragm in mothballs, my clockwork-predictable period missed its due date. For the first time in what would become a numbing pattern, Ed revealed a precisely calibrated dose of superstition disguised as caution that overpowered my garden-variety rationality. To my way of thinking, you'd rush to take a home pregnancy test the minute your period was delayed, but in his weird bargain with the fates, he insisted that we wait a full week. So I bought a pink First Response kit early in the week and placed it on the bathroom counter, where it sat until Saturday morning.

Friday afternoon, while I'm shopping at B. Altman's on Fifth Avenue, I begin to spot. I have a moment of distress, but then I calm down. My period's late! It's never late! I meet Ed after work in the February chill and we sit through a movie before I mention anything to him. I've already lathered myself back up into optimism, but to Ed it is that first crush of bad news and I can't bear the new look on his face. All week he'd been hounding me like an excited puppy hoping for a cherished trip to the park: "If your period were about to show up, would you be feeling anything in particular? . . . What do you mean, you didn't have any coffee this morning? Did you feel nauseous? Have you ever not wanted coffee before? . . ."

The next morning, Valentine's Day, we take the test, even though I'm still spotting. In 1987 taking a home pregnancy test was a protracted laboratory experiment. You had to pour liquid back and forth between vials, wait five minutes, add some new chemical to the mix, then wait fifteen minutes more. There were a lot of steps; you could definitely blow it. Ed performs the scientific duties with a serious mien, then we set the kitchen timer for fifteen minutes. While the concoction of my urine and the mysterious chemical substances prepares to yield up its secret on our bathroom counter, Ed and I dance slowly in the living room, with no music, to make the time pass. We try to smile and joke, holding each other close, until we hear the dinger.

And then something simple happens, an innocent mistake, a clumsy mistake, that will leave me angry and embarrassed and will brand this in our medical charts as an "undocumented pregnancy." In his eagerness and nervousness, Ed knocks over the vials with their precious liquid before the final step can be followed. There are a few sharp words, then the heavy silence of disappointment as we acknowledge that I'm bleeding, not just spotting. There's no point in going out and getting another test.

In the shower I can see that this is no ordinary period. The blood is flowing freely down my legs and into the streaming water on the tub floor, as if from a wound, as if from something pumped. I wonder if I am painlessly, effortlessly losing what we have conceived.

We spend the day reading inside, chastened, mildly shocked. By evening I can use the walk, so I offer to pick up some takeout on Third Avenue from our favorite Chinese restaurant (our favorite as much for the food as the name: Fu's Rush Inn). The contact with the outside world does me good. I enjoy the crisp night air and the small accomplishment of making dinner appear on the table.

But while we're dishing up the food, I begin to feel strange in some unquantifiable way. It is instantly clear to me that I will not be having dinner. That morning I had put on a tan cable-knit sweater, and now it seems that whole lives come and go, entire decades pass, while I stare and stare at those neat braided rows. I can't get comfortable, even after I lie down on the bed. A slow arc of pain stretches across my abdomen, gripping me with its sharp, bony fingers. It is a cramp, a contraction, that won't let go. I wind up in the empty bathtub, fully clothed, lying on my back with my legs bent at the knees, stirrup style: my private labor.

Ed sits on the edge of the tub trying to soothe me, tenderly talking me through it. Hour after hour passes. The cramp, it seems, will never loosen its hold. Someone is twisting my uterus, wringing out its juices, emptying it of every moist and warm place where a fertilized egg could nestle. Deep into the night the grip eases a little and I am able to sleep soundly until morning.

By the next day and the day after, it is just another menstrual cycle, and we have no hard evidence that it was ever anything else. But I know I have miscarried—I feel strange and sober about it, more shocked than sad—and I want to be seen by a doctor.

This is what Ed and I are like, or what we became as we went through our infertile years: we expect our experience to be invalidated; we are ready to capitulate to an authority who will tell us that what we know has happened hasn't. This is partly from a hard-ass empirical attitude Ed has picked up along the way and sporadically recruited me into. He knew what I went through that night, but his scientist side knew only that we had no pregnancy-test results. So, his thinking went, why would any medical person invest meaning in a description of a bad night in a tub when there is no colored vial to support it?

But Dr. Singh surprises us. She does not interrogate or smirk. She listens, and then explains that I expelled a conceptus somewhere in that menstrual flow. She names that night for us. I have had, she says, what is called an early miscarriage (at five weeks), supporting my theory that I was in fact in a kind of dullard's labor. "Yes," I say with a nod, "at one point I needed to lie down with my legs bent, as though I were in labor." This she accepts. Then she takes a culture to test for chlamydia, a common culprit in miscarriages, and explains to us what an ovulation thermometer is and how to use it. I am surprised to learn that miscarriage occurs in one of every five pregnancies, and that doctors don't begin to worry unless you've had several. Most couples can be expected to conceive again soon.

There are plenty of months left in the year. Through the spring and summer and fall, we obey the simple morning ritual of our Ovulindex thermometer in its sturdy, laminated white box. Some women, Dr. Singh had said, find the thing so obtrusive as to be unusable. You must place the thermometer under your tongue the moment you awaken every morning, and lie still for several minutes until an accurate reading is reached. No swinging your legs out of bed and into slippers, no sip of coffee; not even sitting upright is allowed. You should try to wake as early on the weekends as you do for work. It is different from the family thermometer only in that the range of temperatures it shows is very narrow, so that you can easily read to the tenth of a point. A woman's temperature rises slightly as she is about to ovulate and dips just before menstruation. Taking your temperature daily enables you to plot a graph to determine whether your cycle follows the proper temperature changes and hormonal shifts, and helps you determine the optimal days for having intercourse.

I am happy to be in thrall to this glass tube. Something is apparently wrong with my baby-making apparatus, and I like having the scientific means to find out what. The thermometer box contains a folded page filled with tiny red charts, ready for plotting the points of each day's temperature. My charts are beautiful specimens: an obvious rise signaling the approach of fertile days, a precipitous drop just before menstruation, each cycle exactly twenty-eight days long. I plot with heady intensity in black ink. Month after month I draw in my perfect chart. Month after month I don't get pregnant.

But something else does begin happening. Sometimes on the first day of my cycle, I feel an even tighter grip on my uterus than I did during the miscarriage. For a whole day I can't eat, can't even do my freelance work at home. I'm bent double if I try to stand or walk. I'd suffered bad menstrual cramps before, but nothing like this. My beloved tabby cat jumps onto my stomach while I'm reclining on the couch on one of these days, and I burst into shocked tears, eyes wide with panic, like a wounded animal. Heat and pain emanate from a tender wound, an internal fire. On the second day of these cycles the intense grip releases but I still feel its shadow, its dull aftermath, the sensation that something deep and terrible had resided there the day before.

Ed is compassionate, but needs something he can latch onto. He quizzes me, as he had during the week before we took the pregnancy test.

"What does it feel like, exactly? Are you in pain?"

"I'm just very *aware* of that area," I respond, finding it difficult to describe what the absence of recent pain feels like. It's not until the third time it happens that I seek medical attention. We are stoics, my husband and I, sweating out days and days of high fevers, bandaging up serious wounds, without calling for help. Ed feels his body is more capable of healing itself than it is, and I have picked up this habit from him in our years together.

But this time I act. It seems silly to haul ass out to Dr. Singh's office in New Jersey, where Ed and I had lived for a while before we got married, for every uterine emergency, now that I seem to be having one regularly, so I take down the name and number of my sister's gynecologist. Janet's been living in Queens, but her doctor is on the Upper East Side, a twenty-minute walk from our apartment.

The first thing I notice as his nurse leads me into his office in November 1987 is a framed poster that seems a strange choice for a gynecologist's office: two or three pairs of women's underpants hanging from a bathtub faucet. Do we need this lingerie reminder moments before we are about to remove our own underthings? Dr. Weintraub's dark hair (an obvious toupee) and mustache and his large face make you think he is of average height or taller, but when he stands you realize that he is perfectly proportioned but very small. He is a nice man, and

I trust my sister's judgment, but he has one habit that I wish some former patient had cured him of, like the coworker who leaves an anonymous bottle of mouthwash on someone's desk: when he's talking to you in his office before the examination, he motions with his head in the direction of your pelvic region. "When I take a look down there," he says in response to the list of your symptoms, nodding toward your pubis, "I'll see."

There is, not surprisingly, nothing to be found upon examination. I happen to mention that Ed and I will be moving to the suburbs in a few months (after six happy years as urbanites), and he brightens, telling me about a facility not too far from our new house where he has operating privileges and where "they are doing wonderful things." He is getting ready to release me into those doctors' hands, but I object. "Isn't there anything you can do *now*?" I ask plaintively. Who knows when we will actually close on the house, and three or four months seems an eternity when we have already been trying to have a baby for a year and a quarter.

I am a woman with dubious motivation. At this point I'm more interested in getting to the bottom of an obvious medical problem than in conceiving. But across from his neat desk this doctor sees the stereotype of a professional woman who is beginning to obsess about having a baby. "I know," he says, a nice guy verging on patronizing me, "you want to have a baby more than anything, but it's only been a little over a year. In Europe, they don't even begin to treat for infertility until a couple's been trying for *two* years." Well, bully for the Europeans. I'm in New York City and I want some answers. This is what I say to *myself*. To him, I say that I'd rather use the next few months to begin eliminating possible causes.

I've already been thinking that I may have endometriosis, which my sister has been diagnosed with—she nearly died from a ruptured tubal pregnancy it caused—and which I seem to have several symptoms of. It's a "benign cancer," according to the gynecological literature, that can cause severe, incapacitating pain, infertility (among 30 to 40 percent of women with the disease), and possibly an increased chance of pregnancy loss. It is estimated that about five million women in the U.S. have it, and it had historically been seen as a "career woman's disease," since general, misguided opinion had it that it was concentrated among upper-middle-class white women who had delayed having children. With improved diagnostic techniques (and the noise that began to be heard from the Endometriosis Association, headquartered in Milwaukee), endometriosis has of course been shown to appear in women of all races and walks of life. Those at greater risk are women who began menstruating young (I was all of ten), those with shorter than the standard twenty-eight-day cycles (not me, with my enviable charts), and those with a heavy, long flow (that's me; I had to take two iron supplements every day to stave off anemia).

There are conflicting theories as to its cause, but endo results when the tissue that normally lines the inside of the uterus, or endometrium, somehow takes root outside the uterus—in the open abdominal cavity, on the bladder, strung between organs—and continues to do what it's supposed to do: bleed every month. Its contribution to infertility consists of either physically blocking the egg's journey or somehow signaling a woman's system with some general command not to perform properly. But its presence can't be confirmed, no matter how many symptoms you have, without invasive surgery. And it's too early in our travels for that.

Dr. Weintraub relents and explains that the initial work-up, once Ed's semen is tested and found to pass muster (which it does), would be for me to undergo a hysterosalpingogram, a ridiculously oversyllabled word that doctors often jauntily shorten to hysterogram. In this standard first step in evaluating a woman's reproductive chances, dye is injected through the cervix—that doughnut-shaped mound between the vagina and the womb—and an X ray is taken as it fills the uterine cavity to reveal any blockages. There is a highly respected doctor in town he can refer me to so that I needn't wait until we relocate to continue our search for the cause of the infertility and the pain.

I see this bear of a man the following month—I'll call him Dr. Baer. He is the third doctor I have come to this year for loin-related help. I'm not fussy or obsessive, but something's clearly wrong, and I want a doctor to tell me what it is. In a preliminary visit in his office, Dr. Baer explains what will happen during the hysterogram. He is not exactly leering, but he seems way too chipper about performing the procedure on me. Apparently his office is dry or overheated, because I become peculiarly aware of the contour of my hard contact lenses. Moments later one pops out onto my shirt, and I fiddle with it while he watches me, bemused. When I get up to leave, he throws his huge arms around me and tells me he likes me. I can't tell whether he's just full of himself and enjoys giving 'grams to young women, or whether I am behaving in a manner that has touched something in him.

I fill out some forms using my one good eye, cupping my expelled lens in my free hand, while a nurse gives me a date and time for the hysterogram. I am told to expect some cramping as the dye makes its way through the uterus (I've heard from some women that it's a pretty painful process, though mercifully short) and to plan on taking it easy the rest of the day. I steel myself, hoping for some real information to come out of it, but fearless at the prospect of the procedure.

On the morning of the hysterogram, the staff is so kind and friendly that I am tossed into nervousness. They will be mucking around doing their jobs in half an hour; *I'll* be having dye poured into my sanctum sanctorum and paying for radioactive pictures to be taken of it. (My copy of *Our Bodies, Ourselves* had this succinct comment about hysterograms: "Remember that whenever you have X-rays, you are irradiating all future eggs." I pretended to gather information and reassurance, but apparently nothing could steer me clear of these medical procedures.)

Since the age of four, when my nose got broken by a baseball bat during a neighborhood game, I had never needed any serious medical attention. But this place is a solemn house of medicine, Dr. Baer's lightheartedness notwithstanding. I break into a light sweat, fearing that I have not properly prepared myself. I pull one of the nice assistants aside with a shameful secret. "Listen," I tell her, my heart fluttering, my voice hushed, "I always, you know, *douche* before a gynecologist's exam . . . sort of like brushing your teeth before going to the dentist"—and here I try to flash a conspiratorial smile. "Do you think it's going to throw the test results off?" I have images of my cleansing regimen rinsing away flotsam and jetsam that would be invaluable in my diagnosis, rendering the whole painful thing moot.

The young woman smiles in reassurance. It has probably never occurred to her to brush her teeth before seeing the dentist. To her I am a fastidious fool, probably a colon irrigator. "Why don't you just wait for the doctor?" she asks through her smile. Soon my hygiene fears will seem comical and sinister in light of what happens during the test: something so huge is blocking up my uterus that Dr. Baer can't get even a small stream of dye through.

I am lying on a large metal table, something that belongs in a meat locker or a boxer's dressing room. A speculum, that metal instrument all women are accustomed to feeling for the few seconds a gynecologist needs to perform a routine exam and take a Pap smear, stretches me open for close to an hour while I am slid repeatedly back and forth under the radiologist's machinery. Dr. Baer and his assistant are quiet, puzzled. "Is it because of me?" I keep asking, fearing that there's something wrong with my anatomy that won't let their fancy, expensive instruments do their work. But the young woman holding my hand misunderstands and keeps answering, "No, you're doing everything just fine. Don't worry."

They apologize. They reposition. They slide me under the device again and try once more to inject the dye. From either the physical tension of the speculum or the mental tension of the belabored procedure, my legs, bent at the knees, begin shaking wildly, spastically. I am shivering beneath my flimsy gown. I don't know what to make of this, or what to say about it to the medical team around the table. I'm stumping them, I'm out of control from the waist down, but I feel an obligation to keep up a running commentary. I want them to like me despite my abnormality.

After a small eternity, the speculum is removed and I am allowed to dress. Dr. Baer clips my X rays onto a light board in his office and begins reviewing them with me, as though I were an intern, a colleague. On a notepad he draws me a picture of how the dye would normally fill up the goat-skull shape of the uterus. A blockage here and there would distort the expected shape, but this, this! Absolutely nothing can get through. "If you were older, say, in your fifties, I'd have to say you had endometrial cancer."

I give nothing away, but my mind freezes around the word. I don't hear anything else he says, except his patronizing, clueless admonishment not to have intercourse for three days. As if I were going to allow anything else in there after being intimate with a speculum for sixty minutes! But just in case it's the Victorian era and I hold no sway over my ravenous husband's desires, he offers me a quote I can use in fending him off: "Dr. Baer says no!" This line he delivers with his arm once again thrown around me, his massive head in my face, his finger wagging. The official test results would be given to Dr. Weintraub, and I was supposed to follow up later that week.

I took the bus home in a daze. I was the same person, but some psychic and corporeal innocence had been left behind in that doctor's office. I was someone whose uterus was chockablock full of something that sure as hell wasn't a baby. I had sat in a doctor's office and heard the word "cancer" chummily offered. There was no going back. Baby or no baby, I was a patient, and I sensed that I would be for some time.

I was also a wife. Over the years, as the problems mounted, Ed and I would analyze every detail with each other, from every angle, but this was early in the game. I didn't want to cause him needless worry. In a few days I'd know whether or not there was anything malignant in my uterus, so I didn't see the point in dragging him through that particular hell with me.

There was nothing to do but wait until I could see Weintraub. The days were cold and busy, but one dark evening, home alone on the tenth floor of our high-rise while Ed worked late, I curled up on the couch with my face to the wall and shed tears of pure fear.

My fear—well, *this* fear, anyway—was short-lived. I didn't have cancer. I had some kind of blockage that required a D and C, for dilatation and curettage, a scraping out of the uterus. I ask the nurses in Dr. Weintraub's office why Dr. Baer would have casually dropped a bombshell like that. They look nervous, hesitant. "Maybe because of fear of malpractice?" one of them suggests, and I nod as though this makes sense to me. I should be angry, but I'm still trying on my persona as a medical patient, and it doesn't include rage. Just confusion.

It is mid-December, but I don't want to wait until after the holidays for this simple outpatient procedure. Dr. Weintraub says he can schedule me for December 22, and I sign up. He likes to perform his surgeries in the suburban facility he had recommended to me rather than in a city hospital. His apartment building's not far from mine, and he offers to drive me there, the only catch being that I'll have to wait the whole morning until his other procedures are finished for my ride back. I'm so astonished at this scenario that I say yes to all of it. His nurse calls to confirm, and I mentally prepare for my first operation. I still have my tonsils, I still have my appendix, and I still have my reproductive organs, for what they're worth.

I feel hopeful, buoyant, as the doctor picks me up on my street corner. For some reason I have sort of dressed up for the occasion, in a checked skirt and matching blouse. (Even odder is that now, ten years later, I remember what I wore for a D and C! The spectacle of my infertility was beginning to play itself out like a bad home movie.) Dr. Weintraub leans across to open the passenger door, and I bounce in, hair washed, legs shaved, as if I'm being interviewed, not operated on, for my candidacy for motherhood. I was nervous that morning and choked back only a glass of water and half a bowl of cereal.

"How do you feel?" the doctor asks, smiling, friendly, as he pulls into the stream of traffic. Before I can respond, he answers the question himself: "Hungry?" When I frown in confusion, he has a moment of concern. "My nurse told you not to eat or drink anything, right?" "Uh, no," I sputter, already flunking my first surgery before I get anywhere near the O.R. He is not angry or arrogant. "She must have thought I told you, and I assumed *she* did," he says apologetically. "I can still do the D and C, but I won't be able to put you out completely. Do you want to reschedule?"

I still can't believe he's chauffeuring me to my operation—there's no way I'm going to make him cancel it. Besides, I want to get it over with before Christmas. During the drive we begin to chat about my sister, who's been his patient for a while, and soon I find myself telling him inappropriate family stories while staring at a bottle of pain reliever between us. Somehow I feel he knows Janet to the core, although she has probably had but a few checkups with him. He is the all-knowing, all-curing medical man, and I am helpless before him. Mercifully, he is able to shift the topic toward a discussion of his wife's interest in French, a love of mine as well, and a solution to the dark turn the conversation was taking. In half an hour we pull into the parking lot of a two-tone stucco building, and I follow my doctor inside.

This is clearly his milieu. Everyone knows him and likes him. He is waved at, smiled at. Unlike the situation in his cramped Manhattan office, he has room here to walk down long hallways, greet familiar faces in passing. His small frame relaxes and expands to fill the larger quarters. He leaves to change into his scrubs after explaining that since I'll have to wait a bit for my procedure, I may as well take advantage of the time by having a laminaria inserted. He seems surprised when I have no idea what this is, and explains that it's a seaweed derivative that will slowly expand the opening to my cervix for the doctor's instrument.

I'm impressed that Dr. Weintraub has come up with some benefit to my having to sit in the waiting room for two or three hours, and I'm certainly warming to the idea of a natural seaweed stretch rather than the blunt force of metal. (When we visit Ed's family in the Southwest for Christmas seven years later, I will keep calling the paper bags filled with sand and candles "laminaria" instead of "luminaria." By then I will be intractably infertile, and will give myself away at every turn.)

But the procedure of getting the laminaria into my cervix, now *this* hurts. A kindly aide grips my hand while the nurse does her best not to inflict pain. But there it is: a sharp, prolonged pinch deep inside me. Hey, who asked for this goddamn wacko alternative? I wouldn't have accepted it if I'd known it would hurt.

Soon I am back in the waiting room in my checked outfit, reading, looking preposterously forward to my stint in the operating room. Then I surprise myself with a sneeze. Not your run-of-the-mill sneeze, but the kind that nearly catapults you out of your seat. The laminaria, I am sure, has been wholly ejected after this violent act, and I retreat to the bathroom expecting to find spiky strands of seaweed lining my underwear. I am relieved—all is intact.

In good time it is my turn, and I am led into a locker-lined room where I am told to leave everything of mine and to emerge in paper gown, cap, and booties. I am momentarily alarmed at being asked to leave my handbag in an unlocked locker—I live in New York and the self-protective mechanism is hard to bypass—but I get caught up in following directions. I enter the room where Dr. Weintraub will scrape out my uterus, and I lie down on the operating table. There seems to be an army of nurses talking, laughing, discussing New Year's Eve plans, trying to josh with me. One of them asks me if I had anything to eat that morning. "Cereal and water," I reply, accurately and misleadingly. By her face I see she is picturing me holding a bowl of cornflakes under the faucet. I stammer in explanation, but she interrupts: "Honey, you had a *meal*. You're gonna get a real light anesthesia today." Okay. Whatever. Let's just get going.

The nurses get in position around the table. The anesthetist puts a mask over my face for a few moments. My doctor walks in when all is ready. He, not me, is clearly the star of the show, though we are all dressed in the same flimsy shower caps and booties. As he gets down to work, I can see only the top of his cap over my draped knees. He is not going to look up at me or talk to me about my sister or his wife or the bottle of Motrin I saw on his dashboard. The nurses have fallen quiet. All the energy in the room has been sucked into my uterus, where I can feel with shocking intensity that a sharp blade is slicing me. I let out a whimper of pain and betrayal, and the nurses soothe and comfort me. It is over.

I am allowed to rest for a few moments, then I'm transferred into a wheelchair and moved to the recovery room. My wheelchair is placed at the head of a long line of women. Hot tea and cookies are being pressed upon us. Slowly my clear gaze and coherence return, and I can see another and another woman being wheeled in, one every few minutes, it seems. A nurse tells me that since I am Dr. Weintraub's private patient, he will come out and speak to me shortly. I am momentarily confused and I feel for these other women, orphans in this place of knives and blood. Next to me is a very young woman with blond hair. Her name is Margie and she has traveled since dawn to be here today, she tells me. In a broad accent, she explains that she is nineteen years old and that this is her first abortion. I don't flinch. I tell her that I am here for quite a different reason, and we smile weakly at the irony.

As the row of women—some weeping softly, all dazed—continues to grow, I finally realize Dr. Weintraub's real business here. I admire him for traveling out of town every week to perform this service. These women are the drama today, not me. I just wish—*God,* how I wish—he had thought to tell me that my D and C would place me in their midst. The products of those abortions lie somewhere nearby, still warm; if only one of them could be transferred into me. When Dr. Weintraub appears before me, I assault him with questions, but not about this. "What did you find?" I ask him. "Did you get everything out?" Like a husband whose wife has behaved inappropriately at a party, he whispers that we'll talk about it on the way home. I am grateful that he does not gesture his head at my sore uterus as he says this.

I exit via the locker room, where I put my checked skirt and blouse back on, then wait for him. He finally appears in street clothes, and we are ready to leave. The ride back is quiet. He wants to wait to discuss my procedure until my post-op office visit. I will find out then that my uterus was jammed up with a polyp the size of Ohio. I picture it as a large version of the planaria I had to study in high school biology, pink and moist, its thick roots burrowing into my womb. Now, in his car, I sense from him only that I have nothing serious to worry about.

It is only midafternoon when I turn the key in the door to our apartment, but I feel as though I've been gone for days. Ed's at work and won't be home for some time. Margie will be traveling for hours before getting home. She'll tell her boyfriend all about it—he couldn't come with her, she said—but will never tell her parents. I think of the women I know who have terminated a pregnancy. Never did I picture them in a lineup, abandoned and anonymous.

I don't realize that it's unusual to suffer pelvic pain after a D and C, so I don't mention it to Dr. Weintraub. I didn't expect any aftereffects, or I wouldn't have scheduled it so close to the holidays. The photos of me that Christmas show a pale woman with a wan smile, her hand stretched across her abdomen in a reflexive attempt to shield and soothe it. I am starting not to recognize her.

# Chapter 4

# Chemical Warfare

Doctor and patient laughed, and so did I, but my laughter seemed to be coming from a distance. It was *The Dr. Gold Show,* and I was in the studio audience listening to the medicine man interview his current guest. Dr. Gold hardly noticed I was there, and he offered little acknowledgment of who I was: the husband of the patient he was talking to.

Linda seemed totally at ease with this fertility specialist who had been recommended to us by her gynecologist in the city. She cracked jokes with him, and Dr. Gold seemed amused by her. After two years of trying to have a baby, I was grateful for any levity during the nerve-wracking medical investigation into our problem. I was also relieved that Linda hadn't been completely turned off to the medical establishment; she'd already had to undergo a difficult hysterosalpingogram and D and C.

Right after meeting Dr. Gold I mentioned that I sometimes ghostwrote articles for medical journals, and that I had been a premed student for a while. He seemed little impressed by these items from my resume. But what did I expect him to say? "That's great, Ed. Why don't you scrub in when I start probing Linda's uterus? I'll let you take a biopsy."

Since Dr. Gold's fertility practice was affiliated with a teaching hospital, medical students were standing by to absorb his pearls of medical wisdom. The students never looked at me; I was of no medical significance at this time. All that mattered was Linda, because she probably had endometriosis.

As all medical spotlights became focused on Linda, I couldn't help noticing a shift in her perspective. The word "baby" seemed to drop out of her vocabulary, and she seldom discussed the ultimate goal of the treatment. I was beginning to think that she regarded intercourse as nothing more than part of her prescribed medical regimen, that I could have been any man having sex with her. I never talked to her about these things; they seemed petty compared with her medical problems, and I didn't want to add any more stress to the situation. I also didn't want to invite too much reflection on the difficult track we were now on, since it had taken her so long to embrace the notion of parenthood.

Onc way to deal with endometriosis is to laser it away, then try to conceive before the invading tissue returns. On the day Dr. Gold had scheduled the laser procedure, he began discussing another option, as if the news had just come over the ticker tape on a medical hot line. There was an experimental drug, he claimed, that had shrunk endometrial growths in experimental trials. Dr. Gold said that his clinic was doing a study that Linda might want to consider becoming part of. I felt twice as desperate as I had a minute before. Had Dr. Gold decided that we were out of the range of standard treatments and needed to resort to a long shot to conceive?

Worst of all, we had to make a decision about using the drug right away. If we said yes, Dr. Gold wouldn't remove any of Linda's endometriosis that day; he would just take a look so he'd be able to gauge any change after six months of the drug treatment. If we said no, he would laser the bad stuff away, but we would be disqualified from using the drug. Dr. Gold had traded his white coat for a stockbroker's suit, giving us a tip on a hot stock that could go through the roof or go bust, but that had to be bought without delay.

The name of the drug was scariest of all: Zoladex. It sounded like a planet from some distant solar system. As Dr. Gold spouted statistics about Zoladex's success rate in Europe, where it had been approved for the general public, I felt like we were in a spaceship hurtling away from everything we'd ever known. Meanwhile, the copywriter/carnival barker in my head couldn't help coming up with headlines. "Tomorrow's infertility treatment, yours today!" "Zoladex takes the 'in' out of infertility!"

Dr. Gold believed that Zoladex was a worthwhile choice for us. There was also another enticement: the drug company would pick up the tab during the six-month course of treatment.

What Zoladex did wasn't subtle—it would stop Linda's menstrual cycle for half a year. It also posed a slight risk of something very disturbing, which showed up in a long list of possible side effects on the form we needed to sign: Linda's cycles might not return after the treatment was over. *Permanently unable to have children.* Dr. Gold waved this possibility away with his slender, deft hands, somehow telling us simultaneously that it would definitely not happen and that it could happen.

I looked deeply into his face, checking for a narrowing of the eyes or tightening of the lips: any traces of uncertainty or deviousness. There weren't any. My view of him glazed over as I traveled back to 1968. I was a sophomore in high school and my mother had just returned from two weeks in the hospital. She'd had an operation because a few weeks earlier at dinner some food had remained lodged halfway down her esophagus. As a toddler, my mother had taken a swig from a bottle of lye in the Minnesota farmhouse where she'd been born. The lye had burned part of her throat, and over the years the scar tissue had become stiffer and made it increasingly difficult to swallow. After the incident at dinner, she secured the services of a top gastrointestinal surgeon at a local hospital. It was determined that the damaged part of her esophagus would be removed and replaced with a piece of plastic tubing.

It seemed a reasonable course of action to me, an A student in biology and chemistry who at that time planned on becoming a doctor someday. But that was not what was done. Instead, the surgeon removed the scarred area and hoisted up the rest of the esophagus to reattach it. In the process he tilted the stomach, which from then on would cause food to pass into her small intestine too quickly, saddling her with permanent digestive problems. It was never made clear to me why the tubing wasn't put in as originally planned. Or whether the surgeon had even told my mother about the change in strategy.

Twenty years later, I couldn't help but think that maybe Dr. Gold wanted us to do something that wasn't in our best interests. That maybe my mother had been in the hospital being prepped for surgery when the doctor or one of his henchmen came in and told her, "Wait, here's this alternative, but you have to decide right away." Like many people, maybe my mother had thought her doctor was God, not realizing that he might be a mere mortal equipped with too many facts and too much confidence.

"Is this the type of thing where the drug detects all the endometriosis, like an antibiotic finds germs?" I said.

"Something like that," said Dr. Gold.

"So does that mean it's better than surgery? Because the endometriosis can't hide from the drug?"

"That's right. Well put."

What the hell was I doing? I had become Ed McMahon to Dr. Gold's Johnny Carson. Maybe I jumped in only because I wanted to impress him with my limited understanding of medicine, which I saw as a chance to become part of the action.

Linda and I looked at each other and nodded. This was the extent of our discussion about using the drug. I tried to forget about my mother's fiasco to dispel this new feeling of helplessness, this feeling that forces beyond anyone's control were launching a beachhead on Linda and me. Linda had faith in Dr. Gold, and I guess I did, too, and I hoped that was enough.

So our infertility moved to a new stage. We were becoming a case study, our progress to be documented in some drug company newsletter, tallied up as part of a percentage showing either the drug's rate of success or its rate of failure. But which percentage?

After we agreed to use Zoladex, Dr. Gold performed a laparoscopy on Linda to assess the full extent of her problem. While she was having the procedure, I camped out in the tiny waiting area and stared at a row of mailboxes on the wall next to me. The operating room was close by, but I heard nothing from it. A half hour or so had passed when I heard someone say, "Mr. Carbone?"

It took me a moment to realize that Dr. Gold was talking to me. He was standing next to me, wearing a cloth surgical cap on his head.

"Is Linda all right?" I said, getting up from my chair.

"Yeah, she's fine. But there's a lot of endometriosis, especially on her left ovary. The tubes look clear, though. That's definitely a good sign."

"Uh-huh. How many tubes are there?"

"Two—one for each ovary; come on, man," he said, slapping me playfully on the shoulder.

I laughed nervously. Of course I'd known there were two fallopian tubes. I felt like an idiot for letting my anxiousness make me look so ignorant. Yet, with Dr. Gold's lighthearted reaction, a gap between us seemed to close. We'd become two players on a baseball team having a discussion in the dugout about the game's progress. No condescension, no air of superiority from this guy. No wonder Linda liked him so much; he was the only doctor I'd ever met who seemed to be talking to me eye to eye rather than from some throne high above me. I latched onto this sense of camaraderie, and felt new assurance that Linda was in the right surgical hands.

Then he reminded me that this was no ball game.

"We can laser what we see now, rather than put her on the drug regimen," he said.

He looked at me expectantly.

"Is her situation worse than you thought?" I said.

"No. It's not better or worse."

"But . . . didn't we already decide to go with the Zoladex?"

"I just wanted to make sure you understood the situation."

I waited for him to say something, for captions to appear under him, a voice-over, anything.

"If you take the stuff out," I said, "we can't use Zoladex at all, right?"

"Right. The treatment protocol requires that."

"I guess we're still using the Zoladex then."

"So we'll close her up and start her on the drug treatment?"

"Okay."

Why was he asking me this now, while a key voter was out cold? Was he gathering evidence to protect himself against possible accusations of malpractice?

No, I was being paranoid. Dr. Gold was just making sure I fully understood what our options were—something I was sure my mother's doctor hadn't bothered doing before she went under the knife. But I would have felt a lot more comfortable if Linda had had local anesthesia and could have voiced her opinion again. All the responsibility was being removed from Dr. Gold's laparoscope and dropped on my lap, and Linda was in the clear, too. If the drug caused permanent side effects, I'd always remember that I could have prevented them.

Was I placing my desire for a child above Linda's health? Was I allowing chemical warfare to be waged on her without giving enough consideration to the consequences for both of us? I was too numb to know.

We had relocated in 1988, moving out of the city and into a ranch house fifty miles away, on a half-acre of land that bordered a lake. Instead of high-rise apartments outside our window, now we gazed at willow trees and shimmering water filled with Canadian geese.

"Now *this* is a good place to have a kid," I thought as we unloaded our jammed-up hatchback with the last of our earthly possessions. Clean air, a big yard to play in, traffic- and hypodermic-free streets, virtually no chance of a drive-by shooting. Perhaps the plot had always been right; the setting just had to be changed. Our bodies would be purged of city toxins, the stress of fast-paced metropolitan life, and the fast-talking cynicism of urban wags. We'd breed like rabbits.

In the spring I tapped into the fertility of the land and became a gentleman farmer, planting radishes, carrots, squash, and cucumbers. My fantasy about having entered the Garden of Eden couldn't last, however. Another six months of failure in our bedroom/laboratory passed, and my garden mirrored our procreative woes—my refusal to use pesticides and abhorrence of weeding resulted in rows of stunted vegetables.

But life got simpler later in the summer when I left the ad agency and became a freelance copywriter. I set up a home office in a spare room of the house, got my own computer and fax machine, and began happily taking on clients. Best of all, Linda and I were together all day long, since she was freelancing at home, too.

A new fantasy uplifted me then: I thought that being together so much would realign our biological clocks, so that our most fertile periods would coincide. I was also happy that the drive to Dr. Gold's office from our new house was an easy one, since there were a lot of appointments. Linda hated to drive and had an inborn fear of merging onto the highway. She was not adjusting too well to nonurban living, so I was grateful for anything that made it easier for her.

I volunteered to go with Linda when she got her monthly shot. But she said there was no need for both of us to give up all that time. Perhaps she would have been more nervous with me hovering over her when she got jabbed.

We no longer talked about getting pregnant—we talked about infertility. It became the star of the film, because the baby stubbornly remained off-camera. Treatment for the infertility was gaining its own momentum. Too many people were involved, too many problems with potential solutions had been revealed. We'd created a bureaucracy surrounding our problem that required the problem to sustain itself.

Infertility disguised itself as something normal in our lives. No visible symptoms, no pain, no overt evidence of anything wrong. It wasn't afflicting Linda or me, but someone outside us; it was a disease suffered by our unborn child instead of us. I imagined a translucent baby, motionless, lying almost invisibly in an intensive care unit.

I found it difficult to work during the days when Linda got her shots. I tried to divert myself by watching reruns of a show I had loved as a child, *The Fugitive,* on cable TV. Sometimes I imagined the needle snapping off under Linda's skin, her being rushed to the hospital for emergency treatment. When she'd come home after another uneventful injection, I'd congratulate myself on my vigilance. It was a tactic I'd reclaimed from my childhood, when I often purposely anticipated horrible outcomes. If I formed an image of tragedy, the real tragedy wouldn't occur: an inoculation of sorts. After my father set off on a boat trip on the Hudson River, I imagined a tugboat ramming into him and killing all aboard. After my mother got on a train to upstate New York to visit her niece, I pictured the train careering off a trestle and tumbling into a gorge.

The strategy had always worked. But that was back when my age was still in single digits. At thirty-five, by which point my life was supposed to be ruled by reason and logic, a regression was occurring: whenever new problems arose in the quest for a child, I returned to childhood, where a toy chest of superstitions and whammies could "protect" me. Only later did I realize that my regression was a product of my need to do something for our cause even when nothing could be done.

And because I'd allowed superstition to play a role in this new drama, I half-believed that my failure to summon it when Linda was pregnant the year before had had something to do with her miscarriage. I had delayed us from taking the pregnancy test, but that had not been enough. I had foolishly neglected to consider that we might lose the baby, neglected to form the image of tragedy that would have warded off the real thing.

Within a few months after Linda's first injection of Zoladex, we shifted from preoccupation with our sex life to no sex at all. Linda's new hormonal status had put her lust in storage, and my needs, the way I saw it, were unimportant until we got her straightened out.

I couldn't help noticing that Linda talked about the endometriosis as if it was only her problem, not one that affected both of us. But I never brought this up either; as long as she continued to do what was necessary to increase her chances of getting pregnant, I was willing to put my frustrations on hold.

After the injections were over, in March 1989, Dr. Gold scheduled another invasion into Linda with his laparoscope. My nerves were wound tight as piano strings during the half-hour drive to the clinic. If the drug hadn't done the job, what next? Another half-year of our lives without a child, more ticks on Linda's biological clock used up for no reason.

After Linda entered the operating room, I imagined myself backstage in some play on the night of its premiere, waiting for a cue to go on. I saw myself hurry to her side and whisper words of encouragement before she dropped off. I put my hand on her abdomen, radiating positive energy into her ovaries. Then I blinked and looked at my lap; fact sheets on medical textbooks were lying there. I'd be using them to write sales blurbs for a direct mail catalogue whose tight deadline wouldn't allow me to just sit there and pray for Dr. Gold's success.

About a half hour after Linda was put under, I went to a deli across the street for coffee. Then I walked over to look at the town swimming pool next door. Although it was empty of water for the off-season and dotted with small islands of leaves, I could still hear the sounds of splashing and wet feet slapping against concrete, vivid images from my days as a lifeguard in college.

I'm an eighteen-year-old rookie on the pool staff, sitting by the three-foot area in a director's chair, the canvas cool on my back as the sun bakes my baby-oiled chest and stomach. I twirl my whistle on one hand as I gaze into the busy shallow end, squinting even through my sunglasses at the flashes of light glinting off the splashes. I narrow my focus on an intriguing sight: two white toy boats floating next to each other, moving back and forth in synchronized fashion. Toys aren't allowed in the pool, but they seem harmless enough so I don't bother taking them out of the water. Then I hear a scream. I turn toward the noise and see a woman racing over to the boats from the entrance to the pool. Another lifeguard is running toward the woman from around the far side of the pool. I remain seated, curious as to what the fuss is about. I watch the lifeguard bend over and pick up the boats, which are not boats at all but the bottoms of white plastic shoes that are on the feet of a toddler who must have walked into the pool and turned completely upside down. The child wails as he's turned upright and handed to his mother, his tears joining the streams of water dripping off his sailor suit.

I tossed my nearly full cup of coffee into a trash can and sprinted across the street, barely beating a car that was racing to catch a yellow light. I arrived back in my seat in the waiting room in a sweat, breathing heavily. I felt like I'd been there for hours already, but only forty-five minutes had gone by.

As the hours ticked by, I looked up periodically from my information on "Target Audiences" and "Selling Points" to spin fantasies of an effortlessly fertile future. Sperm would be armed with antidetection equipment that could trick inhospitable eggs into letting them in. They would be like the bombers in *Fail Safe* that flew too low to be detected by radar, whose decoy missiles caused Soviet fighters to race after the wrong blips on the screen.

I imagined Dr. Gold firing his laser and tried to focus all my thoughts into one beam as well. Where my beam should have been aimed, I didn't know. At my wife's brain to make sure she felt no pain after the operation? At her ovaries to form an alliance with the laser that would totally vanquish the enemy? Or perhaps it should have been a ray of pure optimism that enveloped her entire body, obliterating any doubt, anxiety, or depression.

A pregnant woman sat down in the chair across from mine and my body clenched. I tried to concentrate on my work, but her image filled my head. I looked away and thought about Linda lying unconscious, then looked at this woman, then looked away and thought about Linda again. Nobody could tell me how long this would go on.

Three cups of coffee, one egg and cheese on a roll, one tuna and Muenster on rye with mayo, two Yodels, and five and a half hours after my arrival at the clinic, Dr. Gold came out and told me that the endometriosis had been reduced by the Zoladex. The big cyst on Linda's left ovary had lost its grip, and he was able to deliver the crushing blow easily with his laser.

Dr. Gold did more than tell us about getting rid of Linda's endometriosis; he showed it to us on video a week later. A tiny camera had been inserted into Linda's abdomen along with the medical instruments, not, I assumed, for the sake of our entertainment but to make a training film for medical students. "Anyone want popcorn?" Dr. Gold said as we sat in his office and watched the magnified ovary being prodded with a metal probe, then the cyst melted by the crackle of the laser beam. I leaned close to the screen, the trace of bygone premed student in me sparked into fascination. The organs seemed beautiful and ugly at the same time, more chaotic and less symmetrical than I would have imagined.

Six weeks later I was sitting at my computer writing an article on anticoagulants for a medical journal when Linda returned from one of her regular visits to Dr. Gold. She came into my office and reached out to me with her palm up. She was holding a little plastic tray with some blue dots on it.

"What's that?" I asked, squinting. "Contact lenses?"

She had an awfully big smile on her face.

"It's positive," she said.

I spun around in my chair to face her and grabbed her by the arms. I felt as if I might fall to the floor if I didn't keep holding on. Pregnant? The word had been whited out in my mental dictionary.

# Chapter 5

# Zoltar

In February 1988 Ed and I bought a house in the suburbs, beginning to build a life around a child who wasn't showing up. I'd known the house since I was ten—it had belonged to an English cousin and aunt. On most weekends when I was a kid, my family would make the hour-and-a-half drive to visit them. Crossing the bridge that took us off Long Island, my sisters and I would cover our eyes and hold our breath in the backseat; we had gotten it into our heads that the car had to make its way up and down each of the towering steel arches.

The day Ed and I moved in, two years after Aunt Helen died and the day my cousin left for a new life in Florida, I wandered from room to room repeating my cousin's name: "Pam? Pam?" After two decades of visiting her and her mother there, I couldn't simply barge in with all my belongings. I didn't know yet that I would never be quite able to claim the house as mine, or that after living in New York City any other place to live would feel as arbitrary as someone else's birthday. What were all these people doing behind their closed suburban doors? Rattling around behind my own closed door, I could think only

"Here I am" instead of the comforting "Here we all are" I'd always felt in New York. I'd miss the constant, reassuring feeling that we were all, all of us, in this together. We could hear one another's conversations on the subway. We could emerge from our apartment buildings on a Sunday morning when the entire city smelled of coffee.

I became an impostor, living a life of barbecues and rakes, not inhabiting the place I inhabited, shunning the view out my own window. I was still working from home, editing manuscripts for book publishers, but Ed now commuted an hour and a half each way to his advertising job in New York. By the time he got home in the desperately quiet dark, I would be clinging to the screen door like a cat, panting for companionship. My chameleon husband adjusted well. He loved the big yard on the lake and the deer and geese who made it their home. I had gotten used to the notion that, aside from children—and even there I was coming around—we desired all the same things. I wanted him, too, to feel he was chafing, ill-suited to this country neighborhood without streetlights or house numbers.

But from here, from this false life, our baby-making efforts would take on concentrated focus. Downstairs from the O.R. where Dr. Weintraub had performed my D and C was a first-rate fertility center. When summer arrived, I phoned for an appointment and the receptionist gave me the names of the two doctors there. Neither specialized in anything that would help me choose, so I picked David Gold, for no better reason than that she had named him first.

On the day of our first appointment with him, Ed and I drove into the parking lot of the two-tone stucco building. There was no real waiting room, just half a dozen chairs wedged between the mailboxes and a corn plant. The doctor himself came out to greet us and shake our hands—a courtly, unexpected gesture—and apologized sincerely for having made us wait. I glanced at my watch and saw that it was no more than seven or eight minutes past our appointment time.

He led us into his office, explaining that since it was part of a teaching hospital, there would be some students sitting in. I shrugged and shot a glance toward Ed. We were beleaguered, submissive. It wouldn't have occurred to us that we might have had the right to refuse this public display of our reproductive malfunction.

The questions Dr. Gold proceeded to ask us should have been given to me on a written form. How many women are going to answer truthfully in front of a doctor and some gawky medical students when asked how often she and her husband have intercourse (never as much as you think other couples do), or whether she ever feels pain during it (I did sometimes, but I didn't want Ed to know).

After completing our family and medical history, Dr. Gold led us into the ultrasound room to take a look at my innards right then and there. It would be the first of many, many ultrasound sessions in that room. I'd had the kind for which you had to down quarts of water and have a microphone-shaped pad glided over your belly. For this one, no water drinking was required, but the long ultrasound device would be inserted vaginally.

He called a day or two later with his assessment. The ultrasound film showed spots that were consistent with endometriosis. I silently cheered. At last there would be a diagnosis and a treatment.

"You have scattered bits of tissue, with a very large piece covering your left ovary, and its rough appearance suggests endometrial growth," he explained.

"Could it have caused the miscarriage?" I asked.

"Doubtful. But it might explain why you're taking so long to get pregnant."

"Okay, so how do you get it out of there?"

"Well, surgery is the only way to diagnose for sure, and during the surgery we could remove it with lasers."

"When can I be scheduled for surgery?"

Dr. Gold laughed. "Most patients need time to think—"

"Look, Dr. Gold," I interrupted. "I'm thirty-two years old. It's taken me two years to hear a doctor say he thinks he knows why I can't get pregnant. Let's just get on with it."

"All right. I suppose I could give you a laparoscopy on Thursday or Friday."

"Yes, please. Let's schedule it."

I knew a little about laparoscopy and a lot about why I wanted to forge ahead. In other words, I had no idea what I was in for.

There were forms to fill out, blood to be drawn, pamphlets to be read. Ed and I showed up at the clinic Friday morning for the outpatient procedure and were briefed by Dr. Gold. I liked him. He was down-to-earth. He talked fast and moved in quick, jerky motions, like a shorebird. He wasn't particularly tall, but his legs were long. His face was small and square and supported a pair of black wire glasses and a black mustache. He struck me as irreverent, as someone who would cut through the bullshit and stay on my side. I could tell he was going to let me break the rules. I kept popping back into his office from the waiting room to ask another question about the surgery. On one of these trips, I backed off when I found his office suddenly full of people. "We suspect this to be a case of endometriosis," I heard him explain to them. I guessed that there would be lots of students' eyes peering at me after I was put under, but I didn't really care. Some part of me seemed almost to enjoy the attention.

I would be having a diagnostic laparoscopy, in which small incisions would be made in my navel and at the pubic hairline, through which instruments would be inserted to view the pelvic region and assess any visible endometrial growths. Later I would learn that carbon dioxide is pumped in to move your pesky intestines out of the way and give the doctor plenty of room to see. So, questing for pregnancy, I would appear bloated, pregnant, while Dr. Gold peered and zapped.

The laparoscopy revealed moderate endometriosis (as opposed to mild or severe), and he stitched my skin back up a couple of hours later. I came to in a fog. I had been cut, filled with air, investigated, filmed, and moved to a different room. It was a leap of faith to imagine that I could have gotten there since earlier that morning, when I had walked into the operating room and simply lain down on the table, watching the moon-faced anesthesiologist who inserted a needle into the back of my hand. My head was heavy with confusion and sedation, but I talked briefly with Dr. Gold before Ed came to sit by my side while I revived. He looked guilty and concerned, asked what he could think to ask the doctor. I was a spectacle, propped in a bed with a head full of cotton.

Later that afternoon, at home, I began to feel a bothersome pressure up by my right shoulder. The air that had been pumped in needed somewhere to go. It rose and got trapped there. Ed brought sandwiches into the living room, where I reclined, trying to keep still and fighting to get back to the body and psyche I knew as mine. After a few bites of lunch, it began. I am, it turns out, one of those people who react to general anesthesia by retching. The soreness and surrealness are not enough. No, I've got to beeline to the bathroom five, six, seven times—I lost count—to vomit out the poisons I'd paid good money to have released into my system.

Because of the site of the incision, I was left with a new belly button instead of a scar. I had always had a flat pinwheel for a navel, family legend claiming it was because my umbilical cord had taken a long time to fall off, but now I had a decided "innie." There were two red lines at the top of the pubic hairline that would become part of my abdominal landscape for a couple of years, then fade and eventually vanish. During my post-op checkup, the nurse told me that it was still to be determined whether I would be getting a newfangled experimental drug or the old standby, Danazol, with its proven effectiveness to shrink endometrial growths and known side effects of weight gain, increased hair growth, and acne.

I win the crapshoot: I will be going to the fertility clinic once a month for six months to have a pellet of Zoladex deposited into my belly through a nine-inch needle. The drug shuts down the menstrual cycle, upon which the endo feeds, and so the growths are expected to disappear. (What I don't know is that my breasts and my libido are also about to disappear.) Ed and I find the drug's name cumbersome and difficult to remember. "Zoltar," we call it instead, after the name of the mechanical carnival genie that the Tom Hanks character makes his wish on in the movie *Big*. Careful what you wish for.

I am asked to arrive at the clinic for my first injection on a Sunday morning. These things have to be strictly regulated according to the menstrual cycle, but the effect is that I am engaged in something clandestine: my doctor is showing up on a Sunday to treat me. Elaborate files are made up with my name on them. Questions, forms, in triplicate. Finally I'm ushered into the examination room and told to lie down. No removal of clothing, no paper gown. I simply loosen my pants and reveal the blank readiness of my abdomen. Dr. Gold bounces in, his energy bringing the room to life. A spot on my abdomen is swathed in alcohol, and a topical anesthetic is applied. I look away, as I always do when a needle makes its appearance. As he pulls it back out from my tender insides, Dr. Gold asks me if I felt anything.

"No," I say.

"It's amazing, isn't it? Look at this thing," he says, brandishing a very, very long needle over me.

"You had to show me!" I say in mock complaint. "Why on earth would you think that I would want to see this thing?" He gives me a gentle smile.

"So now I'm going to be like a sixty-year-old woman?" I ask him. I picture Zoltar hurtling me into a postmenopausal state. I will experience what I wasn't meant to see for decades yet. I will be wise, or at least wizened, before my time. But I am at the wrong end of the scale.

"No, Linda," Dr. Gold explains, "it's more like going back to before you began to menstruate. You'll be a kid again!"

I can't decide whether this is better. I rather like the idea of getting a glimpse of myself as a dowager; I already know what I was like at nine. As I sit up Dr. Gold puts out a chivalrous hand to help. It is a simple gesture. I like the way it makes me feel. That it has come from a medical person whose usual view of me is from between the stirrups, who has inserted vaginal ultrasound wands into me, and who is responsible for the current look of my navel lends it a peculiar power I don't yet know how to interpret. He's in this with me, though, that much I know. He has something at stake, too.

I had a standing appointment with Dr. Gold every fourth Monday at 9:30. The clinic had to keep meticulous records for the pharmaceutical company that manufactured Zoltar, draw blood from me, test my urine, and, of course, administer the shot. When possible side effects were reviewed with me, I didn't flinch. Things were gaining momentum, and I wasn't about to get in the way. Besides, it felt good to be doing something about the infertility.

Midway through the six-month experiment there were signs that I was not quite myself. I didn't notice the gradual onset of change, only when it reached critical mass. A blouse that had been tight across the chest now fit with room to spare. The cups of my bra sank in on themselves, puckered and deflated. At nine years of age I had been hiding the fact that I needed to wear a bra. Now, at thirty-two, I wished I had more need for one.

I was changing on the inside, too. In Dr. Gold's office one Monday morning I began talking to him about what the drug was doing to my sense of femininity. I wasn't sure where my talks with him were supposed to begin and end, but he was patient and easy to talk to. And he seemed to be able to give me as much time as I wanted.

"I've never felt very feminine," I told him, "you know, because I'm so big. But wherever you are along that continuum, the drug finds you and gets you." He listened thoughtfully.

"I'm sorry," I spurted out. "You're not my psychiatrist."

"It's all right, really. I'd rather you talk to me than to a psychiatrist," he said from across his desk. "Some people come in and out of here and I don't have any idea what they're going through. Really, I want you to talk to me about it."

As I continued I suddenly became aware that I was close to weeping, and I let the tears come. Through them I talked to Dr. Gold about what would happen if the Zoladex didn't help me. He mentioned in vitro fertilization. The little I knew about this exotic high-tech option convinced me I would never go that far. It was intrusive, expensive, and not very likely to work. He also said something about adoption not always being an easy alternative, but I had a vague assumption that it would be our emergency backup plan and let this comment evaporate into the air.

"I feel guilty," I told him. "I know that a lot of women with endo are in much more pain than I am. I'm one of the lucky ones, but I still feel sorry for myself. Nothing's really wrong with me!"

I had never come across a doctor who listened to me so intently, and I told him so. His black hair was spotted with gray; I put him in his early forties. "Got any kids yourself?" I suddenly asked. It had never occurred to me before that moment to picture him outside his office. "Yeah. Two boys. Sometimes we joke that our patients should take our kids home for a weekend to see what they're in for."

I burst out of the cocoon of warmth and understanding he had wrapped me in. Did fertile people think we wanted *their* kids? Did they think we'd be dissuaded from becoming parents after seeing how noisy and messy kids could be? Boy, that parenthood stuff's not for me after all, Doc! Thank God I saw the light now! No, they couldn't imagine what it was like to try to get pregnant and fail, and I hated them at times for that. An old friend of mine unwittingly sent me a birthday card one year featuring the Little Old Woman Who Lived in a Shoe. I was stunned, yet I understood at a very basic level that I might have done the same thing if the situation were reversed, that she would never be able to connect my infertility to this character with so many children she didn't know what to do. I was deeply offended by a nursery rhyme character, for God's sake.

I remained very fond of Dr. Gold, though. He was my second partner in this. I started to think of him as an older brother, someone who would look out for me, get me the best deals. It was like having a friend who was a judge or an uncle in the carpet business. After that long, teary session in his office, I took on a new status with him. When I arrived for one appointment, the compact row of chairs in the waiting room was filled. Patients spilled out onto the stairwell, stood by the corn plant, paced along the mailboxes. Within seconds a nurse beckoned me in from the crowd.

Another time my Monday appointment fell the day after Christmas and an emergency surgery had been scheduled for someone, but no one in the office had thought to call me. A nurse came out to tell me that I would have to come back in the afternoon. Dr. Gold appeared, too, apologetic. I reached for my coat on the rack. "How far away do you live?" she asked me. I'd made the drive enough times that I didn't answer her question with "Half an hour" or "Not too far." No, it was thirty-five minutes. If it had been thirty-eight, I'd have said so. I could have made the drive blindfolded at that point: onto the winding, narrow-laned parkway, curving around its bends, the hilly terrain around me sometimes shrouded in mist, reminding me of my year-abroad travels in Europe.

Dr. Gold decided to squeeze me in that day, and led me into the exam room where they drew the blood. He sat on a sliding stool and began to prepare a syringe.

"You're going to take the blood yourself?" I asked. This was usually the nurse's job.

"For *you,* anything," he said, in his best exaggerated Jewish voice. They were intimate, these moments, without being personal. His fingers on the delicate, translucent skin inside my elbow to feel for a vein, the insertion of a needle to extract my bodily fluid, a white square of gauze placed discreetly over the wound as I bent my arm up to stanch the blood.

"How was your Christmas?" he asked, his small fingers working expertly. "Okay," I said, and asked him about his holiday. "Oh, you don't want to know," he said. "I was cooped up." I didn't respond, not being sure whether that had been an invitation or a roadblock. And in that rushed session, squeezed in while a surgical patient awaited his healing touch, I didn't bother telling him what had happened over Christmas.

Zoltar had begun to take its toll. If it was going to get rid of my endo, by God it would demand something in return. It wasn't enough that my bustline had shrunk to a preteen size, that it had become impossible to achieve orgasm or, eventually, even to give a thought to sex. (When we did attempt it, it hurt. I told a nurse about this on one of my visits and she immediately went to work telling me what products and positions I could use to make it viable. I wondered whether, if I'd been a man, a medical authority would have reacted to my saying that sex gave me pain and no pleasure by offering tips on how to have it anyway.) Poor Ed—we didn't really talk about it; we just put our sex life on ice. Zoltar or my self-righteousness—"Look what I'm going through for you!"—made it undiscussable. This was about me and my body. I'd forgotten that it had anything to do with Ed.

He and I had ambitiously decided to host both families—seventeen people in all—for our first Christmas in our new home. The holiday coincided perfectly with Zoltar's victory over my mental state. If everything went along smoothly, I'd be fine, but the slightest problem would hurl me over the edge. I didn't know at the time to describe it this way, though. All I knew was that while we were preparing the roast beast and all the trimmings, I dissolved into anguished tears at least five times and had to make a hasty exit from the kitchen. My poor mother thought she was interfering with my culinary plans and that it was all her fault. I don't know what anyone else thought, but it's possible that, with the crush of children and sleigh bells in the house, they simply weren't aware of my breakdowns.

But little Andrea, my sister Barbara's six-year-old, began trailing me out of the kitchen, following me into the bathroom as I splashed water on my face and into the spare room, where I retreated and tried to regroup. She was concerned, she was curious, she was exquisitely, almost unbearably adorable. I didn't know myself what was wrong, but Andrea had heard me say that I'd had to apply my makeup over and over that day. "Now, Linny," she admonished in her high, pure voice, her tiny finger pointing, "if you have to put your makeup on again, it's all right. You don't have to cry about it." I gave her a squeeze and smoothed back her brown bangs. "You have a lot of people here today," she went on, "and you need some help." God bless that lovely child. There was no one anywhere who could have made me feel better at that moment.

Somehow we pulled off that Christmas dinner and got through the next couple of months. I was an emotional quadriplegic, unable to come up with the correct mood for anything. "Zoltar!" I'd announce to Ed when I knew I was overreacting and couldn't seem to do anything about it. "Zoltar!" he'd speak with a flourish when I'd forgotten something important or inadvertently offended him.

A few weeks after the final injection, I was ready to come under the laparoscope again. "It could be a long case," Dr. Gold explained; "come by at seven-thirty so we can get started early." It *was* a long case—five and a half hours long, to allow for the tricky removal of the cyst through the laparoscope—but a successful one. The drug had dissolved or loosened the endometrial growths. Because of the length of time I had been under, I woke up more befuddled than after the last surgery. A pink blanket had been spread across me. I felt surreal, disbelieving. It was one o'clock and I could not account for the morning. Dr. Gold materialized at my side, lifted my hand, and placed it between his two. "You did great. We got all the endo out," he said. "Now you need to stay away from this place for a while."

For the rest of the afternoon and all evening at home, I puked. I was cured.

When I began menstruating again after seven months of cycle shutdown, I had to reacquaint myself with its paraphernalia. Tampax had changed its box design, and I handled its contents awkwardly. I felt recharged sexually after the Zoladex wore off, though, and Ed and I made sure to have sex three times before my ovulation date, as the books and doctors suggest.

My follow-up appointment at the clinic fell a few days before my next period was due, and I asked a nurse whether a blood test could reveal a pregnancy this early. "It might," she said. I had to have blood drawn for their other tests anyway, so I asked her to take an extra vial.

Sitting on the edge of the examining table, stripped from the waist down and covered with a drape, I talked to Dr. Gold. There was a knock on the door and the nurse opened it, gesturing to him. I looked away, waiting to be the center of attention again. "Why didn't anyone tell me?" he said after a delay. The assistants in the office, the nurse outside, Dr. Gold, all looked at one another expectantly. Then Dr. Gold looked at me and said, "You're pregnant." I flung my hands up and covered my face, then wrapped my arms around his waist, my head on his chest. When I pulled back I saw that Dr. Gold looked coy, proud. He was happy for me, but it didn't hurt that this would also make Zoltar's manufacturers look good.

After he examined me we sat together in his office. "I can't deliver your baby myself," he explained, beaming, "but I'll recommend someone."

"Oh, I didn't think you were an obstetrician, too," I said.

"Well, when I first met you, I was delivering babies." He said "when I first met you," not "when you first came to me" or "first became my patient." I told him I wanted a midwife and he wrote down a name for me. "I can't believe I won't be coming here anymore!" I said. I would miss the place, its makeshift feel, its casual brilliance.

"You'll need to come back for some early blood monitoring, but basically you're done with us," he said with a smile on his thin lips. "You'll like this midwife," he added, handing me a slip of paper.

"Good. What's she like? Young?" I asked.

"She's, like, our age."

"Whose age?" I asked. Mine or his? I had presumed a ten-year difference.

"Ours. Yours and mine—we're the same age," he said, smiling. We looked at each other for a few slowed seconds.

I confessed I'd thought he was in his early forties, not early thirties. "We're the same age," he said again. For a moment I was glad my treatment with him was over. I didn't like the idea that a goofy boy who might have sat behind me in seventh-grade science class was now responsible for my medical state.

I walked out into the balm of a perfect April day and drove home to share the perfect news with Ed. I had asked the nurse whether there was anything I could take with me to show my husband, and she gave me a small plastic case that had turned blue. When I got home, I casually held it under Ed's gaze. He was distracted, working against deadline, and only vaguely registered it. After a moment I said, "It's positive." I had waited three years to be able to speak those words to my husband, and I basked in the pleasure of their power.

We'd had one visit with the midwife, and received Dr. Gold's assurance that the HCG level in my blood, whose rate of increase estimates the viability of a pregnancy, was nice and high. But the next blood test a couple of weeks later was disappointing, and further blood tests every few days would continue to disappoint. Dr. Gold didn't tell me right away, though. "I was hoping against hope that it was wrong," he'd explain; "I was happy for you." He volunteered having kept information from me—this baffled me, but not enough to bring me to anger or indignation. I was too fond of him to criticize his approach, but we were getting friendly enough that he'd sometimes fill me in with behind-the-scenes information I didn't really want to know.

I detect that I am spotting one Friday, and I call the midwife.

"Is the blood bright red?" she asks.

"No," I answer. It wasn't. Did that matter?

"Are you feeling any cramps?" Again, no. Later my sister Barbara will ask whether I stayed in bed that day, kept my legs up. Was I supposed to? Was it someone's job to have told me to? Would I have stayed pregnant if I had acted ferociously, like a she-bear protecting her cub, like someone battle-worthy and invincible rather than just tired?

I ask the midwife and the nurses at Dr. Gold's office (he's away for the Memorial Day weekend), but no one will tell me what to expect when you lose a baby at eight weeks. Like drowning or surviving diphtheria, it's something your body must figure out how to do on its own. I'm now an embarrassment to the medical staff, their success story gone bad.

I go to bed early on Saturday evening—bitter, resentful—with the heavy, expectant feeling of the first day of a menstrual cycle. Zoltar has not worked its carnival magic on me. I'm awakened in a dead predawn hour with what feels like a particularly heavy flow. I make my way down the dark hall to the bathroom and find that I have delivered two perfectly intact, slender, glistening sacs about three inches long, fetus and placenta. I stare in slumbery shock before slipping them into the water and flushing them away, explaining agitatedly to myself out loud what has happened, bringing myself from a state of deep sleep to one of deep despair.

In the bathroom mirror my face is dripping, contorted. For a few moments I am alone with the certainty of what has happened. My overriding need is to halve the pain by sharing it with Ed. He will never know what this looked or felt like, but he must know that it has happened. I would give anything to be able to keep it from him.

I stumble back to the bedroom in the half-light of dawn, where I collapse into his arms, frightening him with my unexplained hysteria. A mist is rising heavily, eerily, off the lake as the morning temperature warms the water. Out the bedroom window I see it as a dense cube of fog. The digital clock at my bedside flips to an exact 6:00 in geometric lines of crimson as I grasp onto my husband for dear life.

"I'm so sorry" is all I can think to say to Ed through choking sobs. "It's over. It's over." Now I understand: this had been his, too.

It is all my fault. I have disappointed everyone.

# Chapter 6

# Suspended Animation

I was playing croquet in the backyard. The sun was bright, the sky bluer than I had ever seen it. People around me were talking. I couldn't see them or understand their words, but I knew the talk was cheery. There was laughter. Eventually I could make out my sister's voice, and that of a boyhood friend I hadn't seen in years. I seemed to be playing alone, yet I had the sense that I was winning, that I was playing well, and that there was something at stake.

A cat fight started in the distance, the combatants emitting high-pitched squeals that steadily increased in volume. The croquet mallet vanished from my hands. Then I opened my eyes and saw the ceiling of my bedroom. But the cat fight got louder. It wasn't part of my dream; it was what woke me from the dream. And it wasn't a cat fight.

I turned my head toward the bedroom doorway as Linda ran in wailing. I sat up in bed as she leaped toward me, sobbing; then each of us was clutching the other tightly. After a few moments I was frozen with the realization that we had just lost our second child. The doctors would call it a "chemical pregnancy": an illusion caused by juggling molecules.

I kept squeezing Linda, trying to contain her convulsing body. Her tears fell warm against my dry cheeks. I was too stunned to cry myself, too aware of being there for her to be there for myself. I yearned to absorb some of her pain, to divide up the agony between us. In the days that followed, we alternated outbursts of crying, each of us breaking down after the other had recovered: a relay race away from sorrow.

For a month afterward I lay in the dark at bedtime and thought I heard Linda screaming, even though she was next to me sleeping peacefully. The scream became fainter each night, until it was reduced to a whisper in the distance, a whisper that merged with what I thought was the warble of a tiny baby who was nearby but untouchable. A baby speaking to me in a voice too soft to be heard, unknowable, a shadow that ran away from me whenever I moved toward it.

I had worked so hard to believe in this pregnancy that I couldn't pull away from it when it was over. I kept thinking that the child, or fetus, or chemical compound, or whatever I was allowed to call it still had some identity. As if it would show up as a missing child on the back of postcards in junk-mail packets of promotional flyers, or on the sides of milk cartons. I began wondering for the first time in years whether people really had souls, and if so, whether my child had had enough time to get a soul, and whether that soul would be relocated in someone else who survived beyond the womb. One day, twenty years later, perhaps I'd walk down a crowded street and feel a tremor of connection as a pair of eyes locked on mine.

My mourning continued, still seeming unreal, almost unjustified. I had been spared Linda's horror, but I had also been denied the definitive ending. I had received all of it second-hand, puzzling together my thoughts and feelings from whatever bits of information were presented to me. I was mourning a hole in my future rather than a loss from my past.

Something seemed different between Linda and me that summer. We talked to each other extra softly, as if afraid of being overheard. Although I felt that my love for her was stronger than ever, I feared that I was clinging to her like a trembling kitten digging its claws into the trunk of a tree high above the ground. Had my feelings for her become more desperate than sincere? And if they had, would I be able to shift down to a devotion based on desire rather than need when this was all over? We had been partners in a mostly carefree existence; now we were allies in wartime, burdened with the pressure of knowing that if each of us didn't come through for the other, both of us would be defeated.

Dr. Gold had a simple prescription: keep trying. We allowed ourselves to believe that his suggestion stemmed from medical know-how rather than wishful thinking. We got back to lovemaking, coupling at the optimum times and in the optimum positions, struggling to convince ourselves that we could succeed without a medical S.W.A.T. team storming the bedroom.

With Nature's power to help us and with dubious advice and science out of the picture, I turned to a higher power for help: God. I began praying every day. And I was careful not to be selfish; I always opened with a request that he help all the other suffering people in the world.

Sharing my problem with the Almighty, an entity I wasn't even sure I believed in, was a lot easier for me than sharing it with anyone on earth. I had yet to discuss the infertility with a single person who wasn't medically involved. It wasn't in my nature to air my problems. I had never been comfortable with people's sympathy, anyway. I thought it weakened me somehow, or was a kind of jinx. These were not healthy attitudes, I knew, but I lacked the energy or motivation to dig below the surface for their deeper meaning.

When my parents announced that they'd be coming east to visit from New Mexico, I decided that it was time to break my vow of secrecy. I was certain they'd been wondering why Linda and I, after seven years of marriage, were still childless. They might have thought that we were purposely delaying having kids, or didn't want them at all. It no longer seemed fair to keep them wondering.

As I drove out to the airport to pick them up, I thought back to when I was eleven. My mother and I were riding in the car, and the discussion turned to what my sister and I had been like as babies. After a lull in the conversation, she told me that she had lost a baby girl before my sister was born. The umbilical cord had been wrapped around the baby's neck, and strangled her during labor.

After delivering this stunning news, my mother threw in an epilogue that shocked me even more: I too had had the umbilical cord wrapped around my neck during labor, but had somehow managed to free myself in time. "How come I was okay but the other baby wasn't?" I asked. I expected my mother to say that I must have been stronger, or smarter, or tougher. "You were luckier," she said. "And we're certainly grateful for that." I cringed at the thought that I could have easily never existed. Another child would have lived in my bedroom, sat in my chair at the dinner table, played Monopoly with my sister.

One afternoon during my parents' visit the three of us were in the kitchen drinking tea. It was raining, prompting a long discussion of how it never rained in New Mexico. Linda was at work, and I preferred it that way; I was certain I'd handle the disclosure more awkwardly if she were on the scene. I could hardly talk to her about the infertility as it was, because everything had gone so badly and I couldn't think of any way to make her feel better about it.

"I'm sure you've probably been wondering what the deal is with Linda and me having kids," I finally said when my tea had become cold. I added that I was sorry for not having told them sooner. My mother said that she and my sister had been concerned. Maybe we didn't want kids, they had thought. From there I delivered a *Reader's Digest* condensed version of the saga, telegraphing the facts without any asides about our distress and frustration. Decided to have kids, summer 1986. First miscarriage, February 1987. Discovery of Linda's endometriosis, August 1988. Drug treatment, September 1988–February 1989. Second miscarriage, May 1989. After my summary was over, I realized that I must have sounded like a doctor reviewing a case history. And that I had not once used the word "pregnant."

Then I shifted to optimism, making it clear that we would definitely have a child, that there was nothing to worry about, that infertility was as common as divorce among couples of my generation, that incredible strides in medical science had made infertility hardly more serious than the flu. Later I realized that my preemptive strike against sympathy had nothing to do with them. It was my desperate attempt to convince myself that my situation wasn't that bad.

My mother leaned forward and mentioned the daughter of someone she knew who had had problems for years, but today had two beautiful children. My father leaned back, softly voiced how sorry he was, and said nothing more.

One cold January day in our living room, Linda was flipping through the newspaper, the cat on her lap. I was reading, too, spread out on the sofa. Handel was playing on the stereo. I should have been able to look around and feel serene at such a moment of domestic bliss. Except that I had a tingling sensation all over my face, and my teeth were chattering uncontrollably.

I swore there was an electric current flowing through me, and looked around to see how such a thing could be happening. Had a power line gone down in our front yard? Had a hole been ripped in the ozone layer right over our house? I looked at Linda, expecting to see a mirror of my expression of bewilderment. She was calmly reading and petting the cat.

I began feeling hot, yet when I touched my forehead it was cool. I walked into the bathroom, shaking my head and arms. I splashed cold water on my face. I thought I'd see my body shaking when I looked in the mirror, with all the blood drained from my face, but I looked normal. Until I noticed my ears: they were bright red.

As I came back into the living room, my lips went numb. I sat down again and took deep breaths, but they went in and out of me all herky jerky, like gusts of wind in a chaotic storm. I felt my pulse in stereo in my blood-gorged ears. I put my finger on my wrist and checked my watch, clocking my pulse at ninety-plus, at least thirty beats above my usual rate at rest.

"Something weird's going on," I finally told Linda after a half hour of fruitless attempts to calm down. She put her arm around me, caressed my head. I told her what had been happening, and she suggested that maybe I was having an anxiety attack. Huh? That wasn't something that happened to me. I was stoic, rational, in total control of my emotions. Besides, this had been a surprise assault, and anxiety attacks were supposed to come quickly on the heels of some nerve-wracking event—like when a claustrophobic finds himself in a crowded elevator.

Linda led me onto the bed, where she gave me a massage, but her fingers only seemed to conduct more electricity into me. I left the house and took a brisk walk around the block, taking deep gulps of icy air in hopes of freezing the monster that had taken up residence in me. The scenery was backlit with harsh light that kept blinding me as it sneaked out from behind branches and chimneys. I felt slightly better only as long as I kept moving. When I sat down again at home, the voltage rippled through me once more.

I climbed up into the attic and found the biofeedback device I had mail-ordered years earlier during a week of insomnia. I tore it out of its packaging and looked it over. It fit into my palm and was shaped like a pear, with two metal strips on top and a hole in the side for an earplug. You rest two fingers on the strips, flick on the switch, and listen to it through the earplug. The device works by measuring tiny changes in perspiration in your fingers that reflect your degree of nervousness, simultaneously emitting a sound to inform you how anxious you are—the higher the pitch, the greater the nervousness. While breathing deeply and slowly, closing your eyes, and visualizing pleasant, relaxing scenes, you should be able to make the pitch go down, thereby calming yourself. "Trying" to do this is a mysterious process: a waiting game of hoping that when the pitch lowers, your body will unconsciously keep up the good work.

I came downstairs and hooked myself up. The pitch started high and kept going, until only the neighborhood dogs could have detected it. I had to keep readjusting the dial to bring the sound back within range of my ears, but hearing it again made me so nervous I wanted to flee, as if the device were a smoke alarm.

I had no doubt over what had triggered this anxiety explosion; my unrelieved concerns over the infertility had reached critical mass. The combination of frustration over my inability to do anything, depression over the miscarriages, and guilt over Linda having to go through much more than I did, even though I was the one desperate for a child, had been too much for my composure to bear.

With the grip of the anxiety holding fast, I went through a week of delayed-action insomnia. I'd easily fall asleep at night, then wake up a few hours later as if jolted with a cattle prod, my pulse racing. Nothing could lull me back to unconsciousness. I lay there as my digital clock haunted me with its change of digits from 3:00 to 4:00 to 5:00 A.M., my body drained but my head buzzing. When I got up in the morning, an electric field enveloped my body once again. The anxiety had become a twenty-four-hour menace. Linda told me I should call a doctor, but I didn't see this as a medical problem. It was in my head, so I had to solve it in my head.

I put on my running shoes every day around noon and ran down the dirt road near our house, half-trying to shake the tension from my muscles, half-trying to run away from something that I couldn't see. I got some relief, although the loss of sleep made it more difficult to negotiate the hilly route. I'd hook up with a pair of dogs and we'd run together for a couple of miles, me working hard while the two of them effortlessly trotted in front of me. Sometimes I even forgot about the infertility as I forged on. But not for long.

After two weeks of twice-a-day sessions with my biofeedback device, the storm within me finally began to subside. I worked up to four, then six hours of sleep a night, and the daytime tingling dissipated from my face. I knew that biofeedback hadn't gotten to the root of my anxiety problem, but I didn't care. If I had some other deep-seated emotional or psychological issues, I'd deal with them after we had a kid.

Meanwhile, I didn't like the medical moratorium in our infertility war. Linda's endometriosis may have been removed, but we were still getting nowhere trying to make babies. We asked Dr. Gold for some advice. "I can give you Clomid if you want," he said. "They give that stuff out like candy." Clomid was a pill typically taken by women who either failed to ovulate or ovulated irregularly. Although Linda had no such problems, the drug might still enhance our chances of conception by increasing the production of hormones that stimulated the ovary and the development of follicles, the latter of which nurtured the ripening egg. Linda was to take the pill for several days, starting on a particular day of her menstrual cycle.

Linda's body would be artificially pumped up, and the pressure would be on me to perform. I had risen to the task on countless occasions over the past three and half years, but now we'd *have* to have sex at a very specific time. I could almost feel the hot lights on me, sense hundreds of pairs of eyes waiting to assess me. Within days my fretting had put me right back into the clutches of high anxiety. I tried to rescue myself with my biofeedback device, but the pitch climbed fast and never dropped a fraction of an octave.

When Linda came home from work the night of our scheduled attempt, I held off mentioning my state to her. I still felt that I could bail myself out if I just concentrated enough, and that her concern would only distract me. Part of me recognized that I was thinking way too much about the wrong things. But I had to do what I could to get the job done.

As zero hour approached and my nervousness kept cracking its whip on me, I finally talked to Linda about it. She felt for me, saying it wasn't surprising, that most men would be nervous under such pressure to perform, and that we'd get relaxed and romantic after dinner. She didn't understand. Her attempts at seduction would be useless; only my head could break down the wall.

"You sure you want to do this?" she asked as we got into bed that night. "I hate to see you tortured like this."

"We have to."

"It doesn't matter, honey. We can try again next month."

I knew it would only be worse the next time if I allowed this attempt to fail. The memory of it would expand beyond all sensible proportions in my obsessing head. We struggled to get things going for what seemed like hours, more like a pair of weary boxers hanging on to each other than lovers. Finally

I managed an erection, then lost it as soon as it got strong. Linda tried everything, but I was simply not there. When I woke up the next morning after a few fitful hours of sleep, the layer of perspiration that had been coating me had congealed into a sheet of plastic. Later that day I would have to go into the city to see a new client about a big job. I imagined myself getting a raging hard-on in a conference room just as the meeting got under way.

But after waking I was surprised by a feeling of relaxation in my lower regions. I woke Linda up around 6:00 A.M. and told her I felt ready to give it another shot. She was doubtful at first, but then realized all systems were go. A half hour later I was hugging my ever-patient wife, grateful beyond words that she was standing by me through this.

When Linda told me that our attempt had been too late to take advantage of the Clomid, I was hardly upset; my relief at having done my duty overshadowed her news completely. What I didn't realize was that the incident had become a memory that would haunt me from then on in our infertility war.

A new offensive in that war began taking shape soon afterward. Linda and I were considering calling in the heavy artillery: in vitro fertilization. This involved taking Linda's eggs out of her body, putting them in a dish, tossing my sperm onto them, and, we hoped, ending up with a baby omelet.

Before we got started, Dr. Gold wanted to have my sperm undergo something called a "sperm penetration assay." This bizarre procedure, which involved launching my sperm at specially treated hamster eggs and seeing how many penetrated them, somehow helped screen candidates for in vitro. Was Dr. Gold in cahoots with Dr. Moreau? I wondered, as I envisioned Ed-headed rodents sprinting inside a treadmill.

I captured a semen sample at home in another artichoke jar and drove it to the clinic, from where it was overnighted to a testing laboratory in Texas. Dr. Gold called me a week later to discuss the results. I had plenty of sperm with good motility (movement), but they exhibited poor morphology, meaning they were horribly misshapen: two-headed, blunt-headed, and just too damn ugly for any self-respecting egg to grant entry.

How could Linda have gotten pregnant twice when I had such miserable sperm? And why hadn't my first sperm analysis two and a half years before detected a problem? Scientist that he was, Dr. Gold wasn't going to rely on one sample. He scheduled me for another test three months later. The long delay was required because it took that much time for new sperm produced in the testicles to mature and be ejaculated.

The new test results were even worse. My count had dropped from over 120 million per milliliter to 26 million, and the motility took a dive, too. I started thinking I had some debilitating disease that had literally gotten me by the balls.

With this latest bad news, I could feel my anxiety entrenching itself deeper into me. But what was most unbearable was the sense of guilt at realizing Linda might have been perfectly fertile all along. And that she had been poked and prodded and anesthetized and drugged for no good reason. Screwed-up sperm could even have been responsible for her miscarriages. Perhaps Linda had been wrongfully tried and convicted, and now the authorities had caught the real perpetrator: me.

# Chapter 7

# High, Low, Medium, Rocky

Each pregnancy took a little longer to achieve and lasted a little longer than the previous one. It was like a stutter. If I kept at it long enough, I might be able to get the word out, whole and perfectly enunciated. Being a little pregnant was surely better than not being pregnant at all. It was something.

After two strikes, the world started to look different. I felt as though a parenthesis had opened and wouldn't close; I was trapped within the subtext of life it created. Or as though something had been lost, and I was in the tense, breath-holding interval of the search, the words "Here it is!" already echoing in my head before I could say them out loud.

I lost patience. I lost tact. If people asked me about the infertility, I wanted them to fuck off. If they didn't ask me about it, I wanted them to fuck off. The worst were the ones who told guileless stories of other infertile people they knew, by way of example or inspiration. Or the ones who told us we just needed to relax, maybe take a vacation. Well, buddy, I wanted to point out, if you think it's all because I'm stressed out, how is it that women who get raped get pregnant? You can't get much more stressed than that. Besides, it implied that we ourselves—not our laundry list of known physiological problems—were responsible for the infertility. *Fuck off!*

I was implacable when it came to people's reactions to our troubles. Did this one ask enough questions about the miscarriage? Why did that one flaunt her beautiful children in front of me? Inscrutable but tyrannical, I held friends and family to impossible standards, when I finally let them in on our plight. Hell, I wasn't even meeting my own standards for dealing with the infertility. When it did bring out people's empathy, I was a stone. One young family member and one longtime friend, both single, brought up the possibility of serving as a surrogate for us and all I could think was, "So, what makes you think *you* could get pregnant?"

Worse, I didn't become a jot more sensitive or knowledgeable about how to deal with other people's pain. I squirmed when an old friend talked about her mother's breast cancer. I never brought it up a second time when a new friend confided to me with great difficulty that she had multiple sclerosis. And when another old friend, half distraught, half bemused, told me she was pregnant with a third, unplanned baby, I listened as long as I could, then actually said, "Well, you could always give it to us." Infertility was a good excuse to keep people at arm's length, which is maybe where I wanted them all along. It alienated me from everyone I knew, sometimes even from Ed. Before descending into this secret and shameful world, I hung out a shingle with my new motto for all to see: DON'T TOUCH ME, I'M STERILE!

Because we put off advancing to high-tech tricks or adoption, *years* went by. The white nightgowns I'd bought to wear in the maternity ward wore out. I no longer remembered what baby names I liked. I entertained the fantasy of just telling people I was pregnant; at least Ed and I would be able to bask in their goodwill and buy some time to warrant it. I wanted to be allowed to tell stories that began, "When I was pregnant . . ." I'd been pregnant twice and had some stories to tell, but it would have freaked people out.

So much time went by that even my marriage showed signs of evolution. Ed and I had always been the kind of couple others held up as a model. And we had always felt happy, almost smug, about it. Only he and I knew that we were standing on shakier and shakier ground as we refused to confront the third partner in our marriage: infertility. The partner we consulted before decisions could be made. The partner that claimed our meager savings, as we headed into territory that would no longer be covered by health insurance. In that three-sided battle for identity, infertility was winning.

The more elusive the goal of having a baby became, the more Ed seemed to covet it. What slowly became undeniable to me was never, I realized, going to be acknowledged by him. Simple, painful truths. Our infertility struggle had for the first time made us keep things from each other. It had gotten out of hand, gotten to the point where plenty of reasonable people would have given up the hunt. It had become the white elephant in the room, taking up so much space that we could hardly see each other around it. Although it would form the backdrop to our lives for seven years, we rarely discussed it directly. Ed was terrified that I would decide the infertility treatments were more trouble than they were worth, and I didn't want to crush him by reminding him that I had doubts about making the commitment. He never understood that by letting me talk about it, he'd be making me *less* stressed and thus more willing to continue.

In the back of my mind, I still sometimes wondered why people wanted children. I was a shaky new member of the group. I didn't know what credentials were required. One day I tried to call Dr. Gold and was told he was out of town. As it happened, Ed was out west visiting his parents, and my sister and her family—our only nearby relatives—were away on vacation. I had a moment of unprecedented panic. No one who was necessary to me was around. I flipped through my address book, reminding myself of who I liked. Was *that* why people had kids? The list of people we can rely on in emotional and physical emergencies grows shorter and thinner as we age. We crave connection, continuity, comfort, or just someone who knows us. Was *that* it? I had heard parents criticize people who didn't want kids as selfish, but it struck me that, among other things, having children could be a pretty selfish thing to do.

Nowadays when I think about what got me through those years, I feel perplexed, unable to come up with anything. The word "acquiescent" sometimes floats through my head—the notion that I was just being excessively loyal to my husband—but I know it's more complicated than that. I think maybe I just had a hard time being true to myself. As a young girl I used to endure long, hot hours at the beach and suffer terrible sunburns—I lived on Long Island; it's what adolescents did in the summer. My best friend, Lauren, once laughed at my elaborate attempts to cover every square inch of my porcelain skin against the sun's burning rays. "Gee, Lin, you're really a beach lover!" she said. With that statement I understood that I hated the beach at midday, and never felt obliged to go again. The same thing happened with walnuts. It wasn't until I heard someone use the word "bitter" in connection with them that I realized I didn't like them. Without having these things pointed out to me, I'd just go along with the crowd, leaving my idiosyncrasies unrecognized and unclaimed.

As schoolgirls my friends and I played a jump-rope game in which the turning of the rope would alternately be high in the air, low to the ground, normal, then rippled. *"High, low, med-i-um, rock-y, high, low, med-i-um, rock-y,"* the "enders" would sing in uninflected voices while the jumper did her best to adapt to the changing circumstances. It was good training for the infertility that was to take over my life for the next few years.

In the long breaks between medical treatments, Ed and I always got in three sessions of intercourse at the right time: Day 9, Day 11, and Day 13. Ed had always been a generous, affectionate lover—we'd reveled in ten years of good, varied sex. But now we were fertility patients and sex meant one thing: maximizing the odds of conceiving a baby. The memories of slathering my diaphragm with spermicide and heading playfully into bed grew distant and almost sacrilegious.

Now my husband and I dutifully assumed the missionary position, knowing it most helped the sperm swim toward the mark. As soon as Ed ejaculated, I'd count and recount the number of days since the beginning of that cycle, tapping them out with my fingers on his shoulder, pleased with our well-timed, if passionless, lovemaking. I always kept my knees in the air for several minutes afterward, to encourage the semen to stay put. Invariably those three sessions would be it for the month. We'd read that couples trying to have a baby were supposed to have sex regularly all month long so that there wouldn't be too many old sperm in the ejaculate, but the act became so fraught with failed expectation, even something akin to dread, that we could hardly ever do it without that one good reason. There was nothing spontaneous or sexual about it. These were appointments we kept with each other.

I just kept going with the program, unconsciously looking for ways to make it feel heightened, entertaining. If I wasn't intoxicated by my illness, I was certainly tipsy from it a lot of the time. What made me the most tipsy was Dr. Gold.

I'd become exquisitely aware of the bond that was forming between us. When I got pregnant after the Zoladex treatment, we hugged good-bye in his office, thinking I was on my way to motherhood. He said something too softly for me to hear, but it would have been awkward to toss a jangling "What?" into that tender atmosphere. The unheard phrase and something desperate about the way he held me to him—so tight it hurt, so long it stunned—were enough for me to start thinking about him in very unmedical ways.

What kind of man goes into gynecology? A male medical student is usually a young guy, in his twenties. What kind of in-jokes and misogynistic comments get passed around? What does it do to his sense of women, of women's bodies? Once he starts practicing medicine, every woman who comes into his office is going to take off her clothes and open her legs for him. Is the special doctor-patient trust heightened or destroyed because of that? Does he get so overloaded with boobs and cunts that they don't seem sexual anymore? In the past I'd seen a gynecologist, usually a woman, for a quick yearly checkup and kept these questions out of my mind. But now that I'd had dozens of appointments with a male fertility doctor I'd grown to like, I thought about them a lot.

I'd given up freelancing and taken a job as a development editor with a nonfiction book publisher back in Manhattan. Now *I* was commuting an hour and a half each way to work while Ed stayed home as a freelancer. It was the perfect job for me. I fixed troubled manuscripts, held authors' hands through long revisions, worked virtually alone. It was intense and rewarding work. While I was at the office, Dr. Gold and I would sometimes have long talks on the phone. He was my doctor: it was always okay to call him, and he would always return my call. I found myself doodling his name, writing his last name over his first, watching them cover each other up, no descender letters falling below the line to give anything away. I'd save the messages he left on my voice mail and replay them again and again, the disembodied masculinity of his voice becoming both overly familiar and strange, like a word you say too many times in a row.

I sucked a breath mint on the drive to his office and checked my hair in the rearview mirror after pulling into the parking lot. Sometimes there'd be protesters milling about, carrying gruesome signs and slogans against the upstairs abortion clinic. But usually it was quiet and I'd walk in as if meeting a date.

I was surprised at how easy it was to fall for my fertility doctor. He was a nice guy. He was so *clean*. And he always made me feel I was getting special attention. He was my friend, this man: my sponsor, my ally. I was paying him to get me pregnant—somehow erotic in itself—and he was intimate with my reproductive system. It wasn't lost on me that he and I were the same age but that he was drawing a physician's salary. Occasionally I wasn't sure whether my fantasy was to sleep with him or *be* him.

With a little effort, I could make myself think of him only as a doctor while he was examining me. But had he ever, I wondered, felt a flicker of desire in all the times he'd seen me naked on that table? With his hands between my legs as he was about to perform a pelvic exam or insert the vaginal ultrasound wand, did he ever fight the temptation to linger there, to run his fingers gently down either side and then up the soft, pink middle? I wanted to see him naked, too, to arouse him with my hands and my tongue into a glorious erection. And then feel him enter me. I couldn't even think about it without having to close my eyes and steady myself. (*Yes!* The doctor is *in!*)

I pictured athletic couplings on the plaid couch in his office or in a hotel room with drawn shades and coolers of Champagne. Or the two of us dancing close and slow in a small, dark club downtown, his lips nibbling my neck or pressed against mine in a deep and passionate kiss. He would adore me—my breasts, my skin, my hair. We would sometimes make love with wild abandon, other times sweetly and slowly. We would meet in clandestine places and not have to fuss with birth control. (Infertility has its perks.)

He had everything I didn't: confidence, energy, an investment portfolio. He was the kind of guy who might have broken my heart in high school, just by dating me and moving on, but here, in the context in which our lives came together, we saw each other safely, regularly, under the sanctions of a course of medical treatment. He'd close the door to his office so we could talk as long as we liked with no interruption. There didn't seem to be any medical students joining us anymore, and he didn't seem to wear his starched white lab coat, his name embroidered on the pocket in homey, uneven red stitching, when I was around. Just him in his blue V-neck scrubs or in street clothes. Nothing of the slightest impropriety was ever said or done in those sealed-off quarters. I wondered whether he had any notion of what we did together in my imagination.

I don't think I know of any woman who hasn't had a sexual thought about some doctor or therapist (even, in one case, a vet who had saved her dog's life): the sexiness of his power and his intimate presence, the taboo of seeing him as a man who wants you. But a fertility doctor? Someone my husband and I hired so that we could start a family? Short of getting the hots for a priest, I couldn't think of a less appropriate place for my lust to settle. It proved useful, though, in getting me through the next few years, especially when I conjured Dr. Gold's image during the mechanized motion that now passed for conjugal sex. This was a full-fledged crush. If every hour I spent thinking about David Gold, thinking about going to bed with David Gold, could have been traded for an hour of successful pregnancy, I'd have been the mother of a brood.

I figured that Ed picked up on my infatuation, but we never talked about it. We talked about his awful anxiety problem, about the need to move on to the next treatment, about keeping all our money liquid in case we made a snap decision to try for a test-tube baby or an adoption. Sometimes we took a few months off, but always we returned to the two-tone stucco building. I got accustomed to the routine of my many surgeries: the dreamlike suspension of time, the heavy, sickly sweet odor of the anesthesia, the tentative, incorporeal feeling on the drive home. I made regular sacrifices on the altar of the operating table. Nothing to eat or drink after midnight, just like the rules I followed as a child when I planned on receiving Communion at Sunday Mass. Then, too, I felt woozy and otherworldly, forgoing breakfast for the promise of something greater.

A regimen like that can organize your life for a time if you don't think too much about it. There is an aerobics teacher at my gym whom I love. She works us vigorously and long, and there is one move she favors that I can do only if I take my mind off it. If I think about it, I lose my rhythm, lose my balance. The next few years were sort of like that for me. I was carried by momentum, muscle memory. If I had stopped to think about it, I would have fallen. And I would have taken Ed down with me.

We would know when to stop, I thought. We would stop when we had a child. Though I layered that hope over with cynicism, I began to nurture it and to believe it. We were going to have a baby; it just wasn't going to come easy. We were taking the Rube Goldberg route.

I'd lost two pregnancies. But the way the infertility establishment saw it, I'd achieved two pregnancies without resorting to medical interventions such as artificial insemination or in vitro fertilization. It was expected that Ed and I would simply conceive again on our own. Periodically I'd bug Dr. Gold to do something, though, and he'd come up with a reasonable next procedure. Six months after the second miscarriage (they were getting names now, like wars: the undocumented miscarriage, the Zoladex miscarriage), he scheduled me for an endometrial biopsy. This is an examination-room procedure in which a catheter would be threaded through my cervix at a specified time in the cycle to scrape some cells out of the inside of my uterus. It's a way of checking whether the uterine lining is maturing adequately under the influence of progesterone, to eliminate the possibility of what is called a luteal phase defect.

But my cervix turned out to be extra tightly closed—an inexplicable anatomical fact—and poor Dr. Gold poked and prodded without success. He brought up the possibility of having to skip it.

"Maybe try one more time and see if you can get it through," a nurse suggested.

"Well, I'm wondering if we'll still be friends if I do," he said, looking at me with concern.

Repressing the part of me that wanted to make out with him, I countered, game and complicitous: "After all we've been through together?"

He couldn't do it. I left the office sore and unbiopsied, a case of cystitis on the way. That evening my doctor phoned me at home to apologize for having left abruptly when he was called into surgery. I loved believing that I was the only patient he lavished this kind of attention on.

In the beginning of 1990 I came into Dr. Gold's O.R. again, this time for a hysteroscopy, in which a peering device is forced through the cervix (under anesthesia and with surgical instruments, so my cervical problem did not come into play). This marked the Return of the Giant Polyp, that pesky growth I thought Dr. Weintraub had killed off two years earlier. The anesthesiologist tried something different on me when I explained how I retched all day after previous surgeries. This anesthesia didn't send me running to the bathroom, it's true, but instead kept me in torture: I was utterly, desperately sleepy but could only fall asleep every twenty minutes or so all day, for about a minute each time. I was rewarded the next day, though, with a rare, pure surge of energy and optimism. The drug's aftereffect spurred me to paint the trim in our bedroom, clean the house, and spend $100 on Valentine's Day gifts for Ed and two close friends at work. I felt light and clear, physically cleansed. It almost made up for the previous day's anguish.

That spring I underwent another hysterosalpingogram (not with Dr. Baer this time) to make sure the polyp hadn't made an appearance again. All clear. As Ed got worked on, I wanted to make sure the reproductive machinery in both our bodies would be functioning at the same time. There'd be another hysteroscopy and a laparoscopy or two—nearly ten surgeries before I'd be done.

Ed and I had now been married eight years, trying to become parents for four. I swore I wouldn't do it, but talk inevitably turned to the big guns: in vitro. It was the best trick up Dr. Gold's sleeve and, in his opinion, all that was left to try. Based on his experience, he didn't think our history made us good candidates for simpler techniques such as artificial insemination.

We make some slow moves toward it, including a required semen analysis. The results are "interesting," Dr. Gold tells us. Sperm is tested for its three key characteristics: number, shape, movement. A serious defect is discovered with the shape of Ed's sperm. On the tests and indexes used to measure these things, he barely registers. He'll need to undergo surgery himself. Is the problem new, or are the measurements just getting more sophisticated? We'll never know. But I do know one thing, and it brings me deep shame: I feel tremendous relief at the news that I am not the only infertile partner in our marriage. And as an added bonus, I'll have a break from treatment.

But it's only temporary. Eventually we will plow on, undergoing what they call assisted reproductive technology not once but twice. It will come to an end one day. At that point I'll have a collection of scribblings I'd made on scraps of paper while on the phone, temporary treasures in my wallet: hormone levels, results of semen analyses, lists of questions I needed to ask Dr. Gold. For years afterward I'll carry them around with me, unable to bring myself to throw them out.

"I don't want all this drama in my life," I once said to my doctor. But apparently I did.

It was impossible not to wonder what had made me infertile. And what made me miscarry. Were the two problems even related? Had I been born that way? Certainly no one would have been able to pass me the gene for it. Someone once told me that having green eyes was a sign of toxins within. Were my green eyes proof of a body brimming with poisonous bile, inhospitable even to itself, let alone a new life? Was it our particular pairing that created it? My dear Ed, as I reminded him more than once, would have already become a doting father if he had married someone else. There must have been times when he resented me for that. Did I not get enough minutes of natural sunlight a day, as a newspaper article I once read claimed was an affliction of modern life to be reckoned with? Had my father been right about the source of all medical ills: going outside with wet hair?

Six million couples in the U.S. are infertile. We can't all have green eyes and wet hair. Or have waited too long to try to have kids. But age doesn't explain male infertility, which is responsible in half the cases with known causes. What are we breathing and eating and absorbing that is settling in us with killing force? Are aliens planning the slow but effective destruction of the species, with only one-tenth of us at a time sensitive enough to succumb to their Trojan horse? (Or, rather, their mascot would be a horse wearing a Trojan.) I learned from a magazine article that tampons are loaded with dioxin, a by-product of the bleaching process manufacturers use to get that whiter-than-white appearance, suggesting but not having sterile properties. Microwave ovens. Cell phones. Chemical spills. Tampons. Pesticides. Why aren't more studies being done to explain why newborn fertility practices are burgeoning, but newborns aren't?

I was never going to get satisfactory answers to these questions from conventional doctors. In the fourth of our infertility years, Ed and I uncharacteristically made tentative steps toward two mild forms of alternative medicine. Our friend Kathleen, smart and fun and flirting with New Age interests, recommended a gentle and effective chiropractor. When I called him up and explained my unorthodox reason for wanting to see him, at first he demurred but then he warmed to the challenge, inviting me to stop by for a workup.

He was thorough and holistic, a calming and reasonable fellow with a salt-and-pepper beard. Standing in his examination room, I repeatedly lifted each leg while he articulated my hipbones, making me feel thin, all skeleton, like an X ray. Then I lay down on my stomach, he on top of me, while he made an adjustment to my pelvis using his own body weight. A rather shocking and direct intervention. Maybe my internal basket just wasn't aligned properly to cradle anything within it. It seemed eminently plausible that a swift, brisk readjustment might make all the difference.

As we spoke, he commented on the limited mobility of my jaw. I hadn't really noticed it, but now that he mentioned it, I suppose it did move a bit like a ventriloquist's dummy's. He asked my permission, then inserted a gloved hand into my mouth and bore down on the arc of tissue on the left side. Something gave, like a flexible stick just waiting to be shown the correct position to be in. All my life I had been clenched up, it seemed, like jammed typewriter keys.

"The jaw is the pelvis of the skull," he explained. Of course: a tight, immobile jaw might reflect a similarly limited pelvis. Perhaps both just needed a little give.

I now saw all male doctors as friends with potential erotic overtones. I talked to them too much, assumed a likability factor that wasn't necessarily there. I spoke to them in detail about my infertility, as though it were directly relevant to any other medical problem.

A month or two later I lay down on the chiropractor's exam table again while he sat near my head, instructing me to close my eyes and just breathe. He kept telling me to relax my jaw, to lower it. Finally I told him I didn't know what he was talking about; my jaw couldn't go any farther down. After several peaceful minutes, he had me sit up and he sat opposite me, looking serious.

"It's your breathing, Linda," he began. "Every once in a while you take a nice deep breath, and that's good. But your breaths are very shallow; you're taking way too many breaths per minute. I can help you, but it's going to take a lot of visits and you're going to have to trust me."

I listened attentively. I wasn't sure what he meant, but I was beginning to feel singled out, even if for a serious flaw, and something in me rose to meet it.

"When you were little, you might have drawn in to yourself a lot of pain, taken it in for other people," he suggested, "but then never let it go. But your body knows; it remembers. And lodged in it is the memory of that pain that you need to learn how to release."

I nodded, intrigued. I didn't know what to say. I felt he was seeing right through me, seeing what I had labored to hide and thought I had succeeded in hiding. But there it was, the invisible child I had been: in my breaths, in my pelvis of the skull, in my pelvis of the pelvis. Our days and nights are still with us. Some of us carry them in the hollow regions behind the smooth expanse of our bellies.

I felt as if God had just told me he knew all about it and wanted to help. It scared the hell out of me. I drove home in tears and never went back.

Our second foray into the other side of medicine was with Dr. Chang, an acupuncturist. She had a damp, paneled office way out in Queens. This time both Ed and I went. Ed had a euphoric experience that stayed with him for days. I had pain. Not from the placement of needles and pins in carefully chosen places from my forehead to my feet, some made of gold, some connected to a monitor, but from their pulsing across meridians that were supposed to be clear paths. My endometriosis, I figured, or some other undiscovered obstruction was preventing the energy from flowing where it was meant to. It hurt.

Dr. Chang was an immensely likable woman who gave us little plastic bags of leafy herbal pills and told me to eat lots of beets and spinach, to avoid raw foods the first two days of my cycle, and to boil up slices of ginger and lay a warm compress of them across my abdomen at night. I liked these directions and followed all of them. So did Ed, whom she armed with a different set of instructions.

"I think I can help you," she said, too, after laying her warm, magical hands across my abdomen. Only in the office of someone who's not an MD do you hear such words. "If I didn't think I could, I would tell you. And if you do get pregnant, I can help keep it cooking."

A tear rolled down my face as I lay in the small, overheated room, the noises of Queens distinctly audible through the thin walls.

This is what I want a doctor to do, what this chiropractor and acupuncturist were doing: look at my spine or my knee or my tongue and tell me what secrets are lodged there and what mixture of herbs or food or habits will cure the ailments specific only to me. Mainstream doctors' offices are like employment agencies: they're looking to fit you with what they already have, rather than come up with something tailored to you.

But none of my doctors can answer my questions. Exactly why did I miscarry? Is there an autoimmune problem yet to be diagnosed? How soon will my endometriosis make its appearance again? Is there a connection between my difficulty getting pregnant and my difficulty sustaining a pregnancy? And I can't answer others. Will I be able to move on to adoption for Ed's sake if it comes to that? Do I really want a child, or have I allowed the quest to turn into a metaphor for fulfilling other, unnamed wants?

Lying in the dim room with Dr. Chang, I ask her irrelevant questions without end: about seeing a nutritionist, about herbal remedies, about basic changes in my daily habits that would make me feel energized, up for the task of living.

She looks with patience into my eyes and says, "What are you looking for?" I can't answer her.

# Chapter 8

# We're Looking for a Few Good Sperm

"You've got big veins in there," said Dr. Harris.

A urologist affiliated with Dr. Gold's office had just done a finger dance on my scrotum. Hundreds of millions of my sperm had already been airlifted to the testing laboratory in Texas for three separate attacks on hamster eggs, and none of my samples had performed well. For the average man, 30 percent of the sperm will penetrate the eggs; 15 percent is considered the lowest acceptable for fertility. My average was a lowly 1½.

According to Dr. Harris I had two large varicoceles, which are varicose veins leading to the testicles. These oversized veins brought more blood than was needed to an area of the body whose temperature was supposed to be lower than the standard 98.6 degrees (that's why the testicles have their own residence outside the body). More blood means more heat, which typically has a negative effect on sperm quality.

After the examination I bombarded Dr. Harris with questions. What could have given me varicose veins down there? Was it all those years sprinting down a runway as a long jumper on my college track team? Wasn't it a problem usually associated with women who had been pregnant? Why would they affect only the shape of my sperm, and not the total numbers or movement? Dr. Harris responded curtly to my interrogation: any number of factors . . . physical strain may or may not be involved . . . men get them too . . . it's hard to say. He smiled politely.

During a conference call with Drs. Gold and Harris a few days later, they agreed that surgery was the best course of action. A simple procedure, claimed Dr. Harris; he'd tie off the two indicted vessels. He'd performed it dozens of times, with great success. Apparently I didn't need the veins for any other purpose. Trouble was, there was no way to prove that varicoceles were causing *my* infertility.

Linda picked up the phone while the doctors and I were talking. She quickly took control of the conversation, as if she were my agent in a high-stakes negotiation. She was ready to set a date for the surgery right then. I didn't like her jumping in. I wanted to deal with this new development privately, even though it was obviously our problem.

Memories of my mother's surgery flashed back to me. She'd been put in intensive care afterward, and packed in ice to get her fever down. She hadn't let me visit her there, because she thought I'd be frightened by how she looked. Twenty-six years later, she was still living with the aftereffects of that surgery.

I wanted to think it over, at least for a day or so. "Come see me in my office next week—we'll have a private chat about your options," said Dr. Harris.

So much for "options." At the appointment Dr. Harris didn't offer any alternative to the surgery we had already discussed. The promise of privacy was not honored either; a medical student joined us, and I had to listen to Dr. Harris describe my condition all over again, complete with commentary on what he knew about Linda's and my infertility history.

In the hospital for my pre-op registration, I wandered through various hallways before finding the Admission for Ambulatory Surgery desk. I didn't like the sound of "Ambulatory"—it made the surgery sound roundabout, as if the doctors would be casually exploring my insides—then I realized it referred to my being an outpatient who could presumably walk out of the hospital afterward without assistance.

I didn't like the hospital either. It wasn't quiet and serene like the fertility clinic where Linda had been treated. She'd been traveling first class on her infertility journey, and here I was being relegated to coach. I left with a feeling of doom. I couldn't help thinking that something unexpected would happen in the operating room as I lay there unconscious. I'd wake up permanently unable to have an erection. Or with both of my testicles sitting in a jar on my bedside table.

When I told my father about my impending surgery, he offered me a disturbing piece of news: he had varicoceles, too. He'd been told he had them years ago. But he had conceived three children despite them. Was something undiscovered mutating my sperm?

Entering the hospital bleary-eyed an hour before my 7:45 A.M. surgery, the sun still hiding below the horizon, I felt as if I were about to begin serving time in jail. I had to take off my clothes in a tiny cubicle that had a curtain in front for privacy, then put them in a plastic bag and my valuables inside a locker. Next I had to don a flimsy gown that seemed made of paper towels and that tied in the back. I expected it to rip apart if I reached my arm forward, and it was so short on my 6'4" frame that, if I had bent forward at the waist even slightly, I would have mooned half a dozen nurses.

I was given the choice of general or local anesthesia. I chose general; I had no interest in being conscious of some man leaning his face close to my penis. The anesthesiologist was a nice guy with a bushy beard. He dished out a few one-liners and talked about restaurants near where I lived. Then he left and a humorless resident came in to prep me. This guy turned my hand into a pin cushion; he jabbed it at least three times in search of a vein for an IV, and finally had to be benched by the restaurant reviewer. My hand hurt like hell, and was black-and-blue for a week after the surgery.

The smell of rubber as the mask was put on my face brought me back thirty-two years, to when I had my tonsils removed. After waking up from that surgery, I had expected to be given ice cream, just like in the book my mother had read to me a few days before the operation. I got oatmeal instead: my first taste of betrayal by the medical establishment.

As I started to drift off, the anesthesiologist kept asking me, “You want to go to Hawaii?” “Sure,” I told him each time, puzzled until I realized he was testing to see if I was still awake. In what seemed only minutes later, I was waking up in the recovery room. I drifted in and out of sleep for a while until finally I was wheeled back to the room where my belongings were, and where Linda was waiting to soothe me. I felt a little better when I saw another guy in there who had also just had varicocele surgery; I was almost ready to stand up, but he couldn’t get off his back.

Two days later I removed the bandage. Underneath I discovered two incisions diagonally above each side of my penis. Most of my pubic hair had been shaved off. Linda had been rendered prepubescent by Zoladex; now it was my turn to return to a prefertile, prepotent state.

For the next few weeks I couldn't sit without pulling myself up with my arms and didn't dare sneeze, but gradually I felt fairly normal. I was surprised at my complacency. Valuable time was being lost in our quest for a child—it took three months to recover fully from the trauma of the surgery, and another three for the new sperm to mature—but I was glad for the time off. Even though Linda had reached the critical age of thirty-five—her fertility would now begin dropping dramatically each year, according to the statistical charts—I was nearly giddy with relief at not having to do anything. Our relationship seemed to get a surge, too, even though we couldn't have sex during my recovery. When I did think about my infertility, I imagined my sperm lining up outside a plastic surgeon's office for full-body makeovers, compliments of the new climate zone made possible by Dr. Harris.

In August 1991, six months after my operation and a week after providing another semen sample for analysis, I met with Dr. Harris. His New York City office was near the co-op where Linda and I had lived back in the 1980s. It felt good to be in that setting, reminding me of a more carefree time in our lives. A time when our biggest problem seemed to be how to eat dinner out after work and still make a seven o'clock movie.

Then my pleasant moment plummeted to meet the low pitch of Dr. Harris's somber greeting. He looked down as he led me into his office. We sat and I watched him as he stared soberly at a sheet whose blue color and layout was all too familiar to me. It was the printout of my latest semen analysis.

There had been no improvement over previous tests; the morphology index was in the same low ballpark as before. It was as if I had never had surgery. Dr. Harris offered no details, no explanation, no theories when I asked why the surgery hadn't helped me. He knew of nothing else that could be done for me. I would remain a medical mystery, with no detective assigned to my case. I could almost feel the two scars on my abdomen twisting into question marks.

After the appointment I walked numbly through the city, my usual wide-angle view constricted into the narrowest tunnel, the minimum required for me to continue forward without walking into a street sign or being hit by a car. I couldn't feel sad or perplexed, only hyperaware that no one who mattered to me knew exactly where I was at that moment, that I could perhaps wander the city streets forever and not be found.

I drifted into a health food restaurant and buried my face in a heaping bowl of sprouts and cucumbers and cherry tomatoes that looked more like an exotic window plant than a meal. Twosomes and threesomes surrounded me, their animated conversation zapping through my body as I pushed the vegetables around my plate. I ate slowly while pondering what had happened, and imagined telling Linda. She'd probably been expecting good news, as I had allowed myself to expect after finding out that a cousin of mine with fertility problems had been helped by varicocele surgery.

I thought back to the soccer ball drilled into my crotch at close range when I was playing goalie at age twelve. The 105-

degree fever I'd had at the end of sophomore year in college. The faulty exhaust system that had leaked carbon monoxide into the car I had driven to my lifeguard job in college. Maybe the silent killer had lodged in my balls permanently and was still turning my sperm cells into trolls.

I began cursing the design of the male reproductive system. Why did the testicles have to be at a lower temperature than the rest of the body? Why were they hanging outside the body, an inviting target for projectiles of all kinds? Was that supposed to be a come-on to the females of the species? Wow, big boy, you've got balls, haven't you?

Linda was very supportive back at home, but my gloom was not receptive to sympathy. We held off discussing what this meant for us, that it seemed like there was nothing left to do for me. Then we heard about another urologist who, according to a friend of Linda's, was one of the top doctors in the field. Typically you couldn't get an appointment with him for months, but a rare cancellation allowed me to see him a few days after calling his office. He gave my testicles their first ultrasound examination, then startled me by saying I still had varicoceles. At first I assumed that Dr. Harris had botched the surgery; then the new doctor told me that in 5 percent of these cases, previously normal veins became varicose.

I left the doctor's office with my head still swimming from his sales pitch for some supposedly superior surgical technique. By now I was absolutely certain that large veins had nothing to do with my problem, that my balls were vampires who demanded extra blood and would get it no matter what any surgeon did. And that there was no way any blade was going to touch me down there again.

* * *

Two months later, a couple who knew about our problem sang the praises of their acupuncturist to us one night over dinner. That triggered Linda and me to reassess our medical history. Instead of state-of-the-art medical technology, maybe we needed age-old medical wisdom. After five years of failure, I was ready to consult with astrologists, numerologists, witch doctors, faith healers, alchemists. Anyone.

We made an appointment with Dr. Chang the following week. Her office was a walk-down on a side street in Queens. The waiting room was short and narrow, seemingly designed for children. Then I realized that it was proportioned to Dr. Chang herself, who had to have been well under five feet tall. I felt like I was on stilts next to her. Her child-sized hand virtually disappeared within my grasp, but it was so pleasantly cool and smooth that I felt some sort of healing had already begun.

After a brief consultation, Dr. Chang led Linda and me to separate rooms. On the wall of my room was a nearly life-sized illustration of a naked man, with callouts written in Chinese that were connected by lines to hundreds of dots within the man's body.

Dr. Chang had me strip down to my underwear and lie flat on a padded table. She told me to stick out my tongue, then began touching me gently with her fingers in various places. I'd become Gulliver, pinned down on a beach as this tiny woman circumnavigated my hulking form and inserted small needles that looked like sewing pins into me. The needles pricked slightly going in, sort of like mosquito bites. She kept nodding and saying "uh-huh," as if confirming what she had suspected.

Next she attached wires to some of the needles. The wires were connected to an electronic device on a table next to me, and they didn't inspire confidence. It was bad enough feeling like a giant voodoo doll.

"What's that for?" I asked, pointing to the device.

"Provides gentle stimulation," she said in her high-pitched voice. She flicked a switch on the device and smiled at me as she left the room, saying she'd be back in about forty minutes. I could almost hear the crackle of electricity on my skin, but there was no pain, just a ripple of warmth across my body. Within fifteen minutes, it seemed that my body had stopped functioning, as if I had been reduced to pure thought. I felt nothing from head to toe: an out-of-body experience within my own body, far surpassing any relaxation I had achieved with my biofeedback device. The forty-minute session seemed like hours; I wanted it to last even more. By the time Dr. Chang came back and unhooked me, I had traveled into another dimension. Outside I would walk into Nirvana or heaven, but certainly not Queens, New York.

At the end of the appointment Dr. Chang talked to both of us. She said that we were on opposite ends of the energy spectrum: I was hot and Linda was cold. But she wasn't talking about temperature. She was talking about *chi,* the life force that supposedly runs through the body on different meridians. Blocks in the flow of this energy could deplete certain areas of the body, or build up too much energy in other parts.

I had no idea whether our fertility was enhanced by my zapping at Dr. Chang's office, but for forty-eight hours after my first treatment I felt better than I had ever felt in my life. Nothing could have disturbed my calm during that time. I was nothing but soul walking around, all negative energy traveling through and out of me as if I were an open window. Only this overpowering feeling of wellness allowed me to take seriously Dr. Chang's recommended dietary supplement: leeks and watercress. I chomped on raw leeks between spoonfuls of Raisin Bran in the morning, and grimaced at the bitter taste of watercress sandwiches for lunch. I whipped up vichyssoise, heavy on the leeks, and big salads jammed with watercress and leeks for dinner. Before long, Linda told me that my skin had actually taken on a greenish hue!

By the third day after my acupuncture session with Dr. Chang, the old stress had returned from its long weekend. We saw her a few more times, but I never approached the serenity I had experienced after the first visit. And we remained steadfastly infertile.

Through the years of our infertility, some semblance of a rescue would always seem to appear just when all hope was lost. In early 1992 another life preserver was tossed to us from three thousand miles away. Dr. Gold, who had recently moved his practice to his native California, was suggesting we try in vitro fertilization at his new clinic out there. He claimed that he was getting impressive results, and thought that Linda was a good candidate.

First performed in England in 1978, in vitro fertilization—commonly called IVF—is fertilization of a woman's eggs by sperm *outside* the woman's body. It involves the artificial manipulation of a woman's menstrual cycle, including the use of one drug (Lupron) to shut down the natural ovulation cycle and another (Pergonal or Metrodin) to stimulate the ovaries to produce multiple eggs. When the woman's eggs are deemed ready for fertilization, they're removed from the body and mixed with the man's semen in a glass receptacle called a petri dish. About forty-eight hours later, successfully fertilized eggs (embryos) are placed in the woman's uterus (embryo transfer) in hopes that at least one will implant and become a viable pregnancy.

IVF was hardly a sure thing; only 20 percent of couples undergoing the procedure had successful pregnancies. There was also a danger, if slight, of side effects caused by the Pergonal, such as hyperstimulation, which can swell the normally one-and-a-quarter-inch ovaries to the size of grapefruits. And what about my 4-F sperm? Dr. Gold claimed that, because my samples had always had high *numbers* of sperm, I could most likely come up with enough good ones to fertilize Linda's eggs in IVF. He also claimed that the standards used to rate my sperm previously had been especially strict; my true fertility might be better than had been indicated.

At one time Linda had said she'd never go as far as IVF, so I should have been thrilled that she was agreeing to it now. But my first reaction was apprehension: I was afraid that I'd blow it for us by not being able to produce a sperm sample at the non-negotiable time it was required. I still had painful memories of my disastrous performance after Linda took the Clomid, and a hell of a lot more would be at stake this time.

With my agitation continuing to build, Linda suggested that I see a therapist. I didn't want to at first, resisting with those male defenses of self-sufficiency and denial of weakness. Then I considered the thousands of dollars being spent on the treatment, and Linda's body being invaded by all sorts of drugs and procedures. Maybe a therapist would come up with a magic bullet that would take the pressure off me.

I got the name of someone whose office was within walking distance from the hospital where I was born, which seemed like a good omen. But I began feeling deflated while driving to my first appointment. Now I would always be a person who had *had* to see a therapist, who couldn't solve the problem himself. And what if this anxiety problem wasn't the whole story? What if it was just the first layer of a whole series of psychological problems seething inside my head? I was in no hurry for any new issues to worry about while we were in LA.

I kept drying my palms on my pant legs as I sat in the waiting room—seating for one person only. After a few minutes a man hustled out of the office, facing away from me as he headed for the stairs. A couple of minutes later, Dr. Flexner opened the door and asked me to come in.

He was big, about as tall as I am, and smartly dressed. His shirt was tucked perfectly into his pants, without a trace of wrinkling, and he wore a beard in the Freud style. He even looked a bit like Sigmund. Every move he made seemed too slow, as if rehearsed. The office was very neat, with prints of abstract paintings on the walls. Perhaps the paintings would serve as Rorschach tests, I mused. Three carefully stacked piles of paper sat on his desk around an unmarked legal pad that had a silver pen perched on it.

"Have a seat," he said, waving me not to a couch but to a leather recliner. I leaned back too hard, which made me spring forward again and smack my feet onto the floor. Then he sat down in his chair, which looked to be a state-of-the-art piece of furniture designed specially for therapists. It had two or three levers on each side, and Dr. Flexner spent a good thirty seconds adjusting his position after he sat down. As the appointment went on, he continually made adjustments that seemed to indicate his level of interest in my conversation: leaning back when I said something mundane, craning forward if I came up with something provocative. I half-expected him to launch himself into my lap if I had a breakthrough.

"How are you today?" he asked, after he'd finished nesting.

"I guess I've been better. Otherwise I wouldn't be here."

He didn't smile. Before I said another word he began jotting things down on his legal pad, I couldn't imagine what. *Flaccid grip on handshake. Not funny. Needs haircut. Ugly shoes.*

"What would you like to talk about?"

I told Dr. Flexner about my anxiety problem, the IVF, how I was here to figure out a way to defuse my anxiety over the procedure that was now less than three months away.

"That isn't much time," he said, turning sideways in his chair to corroborate his skepticism. "But I'm sure I can help you."

It took me a few minutes before I stopped trying to lighten up the proceedings with one-liners that he never laughed at. I was hoping he would provide me with specific ways to deal with my anxiety related to the IVF, but soon we were far from May 1992 and strolling around my childhood. I told him that I had been a happy kid, although I'd probably been too worried about letting people down. I added that I still cared too much what others thought of me and wished I didn't. He didn't buy it. He told me that my obsessive fear of letting people down was most likely a subterfuge. I was projecting the responsibility of punishment to others around me because

I couldn't bear the thought of being mad at, or of ultimately not loving, myself. I nodded at this assessment, interested but not quite believing it.

"What about when other people let *you* down?" he asked. "Do you get angry at them?"

"Sure. Well . . . I guess I don't show anger too much. I figure it doesn't do any good."

This last tidbit triggered all sorts of interaction between Dr. Flexner's hands and his various chair levers. For a second I thought little wheels were going to pop out of the bottom and little jets out the side so he could propel himself closer to me.

"People don't always think whether anger is acceptable or not," he said. "They just feel it."

Linda had often told me I should get angry more, that not expressing anger was unnatural and I must be holding back. I was unaware of holding back anything. But the times I did remember having displayed anger had not been cathartic for me; they'd just made me edgy. I felt as if I'd committed a crime, as if I'd somehow be punished for it later.

Dr. Flexner seemed to be on the trail of something important about me, but I couldn't see how his insights would help me get it up three time zones away. I also grew more concerned about the $150 I was tearing out of my checkbook after every appointment. I refused to submit the bills to my health insurance, because then there would be an accessible record of my having seen a shrink. I was certain that such a record would be a strike against me if I ever tried to adopt a child. Linda thought I was overreacting yet again; I thought I was just reacting. After ten sessions, I said good-bye to Dr. Flexner and his magic chair for good.

* * *

My psyche wasn't the last item on my checklist for our California trip. Due to the low quality of my sperm, there was a possibility that none of them would fertilize Linda's eggs. So I decided we'd better have about a hundred million understudies available. I explained my feelings to Dr. Gold, and he gave me the name of a sperm bank near the clinic. I called the bank and a woman told me that if I sent her a deposit—of money, that is—she'd send me a list of donors to choose from. The sample I chose would be delivered to Dr. Gold's facility in a tank surrounded by dry ice.

I didn't like considering that I wouldn't be the real father if donor sperm was used, but saw no alternative. Thousands of dollars were being invested in this procedure, and I needed backup not just for medical reasons but for psychological ones as well. The irony was, I thought that having the donor sperm at the ready would protect me from actually having to use it: a net under the high wire that I wouldn't fall into because I knew it was there.

Linda could hardly believe that I was considering getting donor sperm. She said that she'd rather adopt than have a child that was half hers but none mine. I was certainly aware that having such a child would create an imbalance in the family, with me seeming like a stepfather. But I wanted a child badly, and if I couldn't be the biological father—for whatever reason—using a sperm donor seemed the next best alternative. There was simply too much at stake—our finances, Linda's age, our future, my own fragile state—not to do everything possible to make this one IVF attempt work.

As it was, I was finding it increasingly difficult to consider any of the philosophical aspects of what was happening to us.

With my anxiety continually threatening to boil over, I couldn't afford to add in any more confusion or uncertainty. So I stripped away the emotional issues that tended to hold sway with Linda, focusing as completely as possible on the practical minutiae of getting the job done and winning the prize waiting at the end of it all. It was as if I was applying the principles of my biofeedback to realms beyond their jurisdiction. *Block out negative thoughts. Concentrate only on peaceful scenes.*

A list of potential sperm donors arrived by Federal Express after I had overnighted my check. The woman had asked me to describe my physical characteristics so she could send me a lineup of men who resembled me. All of the men on my customized roster were at least six feet tall, and most were blond, blue-eyed, and of Scandinavian descent. Also indicated on the lists were grade point average and special interests. It was a high-tech version of *The Dating Game.*

All I had to do was point my finger to determine what kind of child might materialize into our lives and become the forebear of future generations of Deckers. Would he or she inherit the genes of a blond, 6'4" art student who liked to water-ski, or a brown-haired, 6' biology major who was into chess? I tried to downplay the significance of this, repeating over and over in my head that I'd be able to produce a sample, that *my* sperm would fertilize Linda's eggs, as I ranked my top five, circled my choices in red ink, and express-mailed them to the West Coast.

Then the unthinkable happened: my number one and two choices were unavailable. Someone else had withdrawn them for their own future generations, and the men had not deposited new samples. My upgraded number one had only a B–

average and appeared to be exceptionally skinny—a mere 165 pounds on a 6'3" frame. I thought about canceling the deal, trying to get in touch with another sperm bank. Then I convinced myself that it didn't matter because I wouldn't need the sample anyway, or that number three should have been number one from the start, or that it was all academic because nurture was more powerful than nature.

About a week before the expected onset of menstruation, Linda had to begin receiving a daily injection of Lupron. Soon after the start of the period, she had to get injections of Pergonal twice a day. Lupron was injected subcutaneously, or just below the skin, with a short needle, while Pergonal was administered intramuscularly with a longer needle.

Because the frequency of the injections made it impractical to go to the clinic each time to get them, husbands were usually instructed on how to load and fire the syringes. I actually looked forward to doing this. It would give me something to focus on other than my duties out in LA, and would let me pretend to be a doctor for a few weeks.

My injection lessons were given at the house of a nurse Dr. Gold had worked with before moving west. We sat down in her den at a glass table, atop which lay two objects that seemed unlikely neighbors: a hypodermic needle and an orange. The latter turned out to be a target for injection practice.

The nurse talked only briefly about the needle for the Lupron, which was very short and would be injected in Linda's thigh. The Pergonal was another story; it went deeper, so the target and technique were more important.

First she explained how to rub the injection site with an alcohol swab. Then she picked up the hypodermic and removed the protective plastic cap over the needle.

"You think you should do everything slowly when giving injections, but faster is better," she said.

She demonstrated how to load the syringe and get any bubbles out by flicking it with a finger. "Imagine you're throwing a dart," she said, picking up the orange with her free hand.

"A cadence makes it easier. One, two, and . . . three." She plunged the needle into the orange on "three."

I picked up the syringe, counted, and gave the orange a jab.

"Too slow," she said. "Faster helps you make sure the needle moves in a straight line. If you move it around while injecting, it could be painful for Linda."

When her young son strolled in the front door, the nurse called him in. He didn't even blink when she asked him to drop his pants, as if he was frequently recruited to be her assistant. She ran her finger along his right buttock to divide it into four sections, indicating that I should make the injection in the upper outer quadrant. Then she squeezed together a hunk of flesh; this maximized the depth of muscle tissue so that the needle wouldn't get too close to a bone.

That night I stabbed a pair of navel oranges countless times, having no idea if my technique was improving as I went on. I was surprised that the needle went in so easily, and that after I pulled it out I couldn't see any hole. For the real thing, the nurse had told me that I didn't need to worry if there was a little bleeding afterward, but that I had to make sure I didn't hit a vein. After plunging the needle in, I was supposed to pull back on the plunger slightly; if I saw any red in the syringe, I had to retreat and pick another site.

Pergonal was in powder form and was kept in a sealed glass vessel called an ampule that resembled a three-minute egg timer. It had to be opened by snapping off the top along an etched groove—an action that also had to be done in one fast, definitive motion, to avoid shattering the glass. I couldn't imagine why the stuff had to be stored this way; I felt like I needed a tiny karate master to break it. Since each powder ampule cost $50 and several were required for each injection, it was important not to send this stuff flying in the breeze.

Next the Pergonal had to be dissolved in bacteriostatic water, which was specially treated to inhibit the growth of bacteria. I had to draw out a specified amount of the water, empty it into the open ampule of Pergonal, then draw the dissolved mixture back into the syringe.

By the evening of Linda's first scheduled shot, I was certain I could have hit an orange with a hypo from thirty yards while blindfolded. Actually giving Linda the shot was a different matter. She was on the bed by seven-thirty, ready for impalement. At nine, she remained alone in the bedroom, as I paced back and forth in the living room while gingerly holding the fully loaded syringe and chanting, "I can't fucking do it," in as loud a whisper as I could generate. I was petrified that I'd hit a vein or artery and that, because I was partially colorblind, I wouldn't be able to see red creeping back into the syringe when I checked for blood.

I was Danny Kaye pretending to be a musketeer, watching my shadow throw one dart after another on the wall. What if

I plunged the needle into the mattress instead of into Linda? What if I picked up the wrong needle and ended up injecting her with OJ sucked up during my rehearsals?

Linda finally came out to the living room, where she found me breathing deeply and doing deep knee bends. I coughed out a few laughs as I saw her, then nodded and followed her back to the room. As she assumed her position on the bed, I realized something: the Pergonal solution was clear. Even I could tell when a clear solution changed color. Any color at all coming back into the syringe would have to be blood.

I wiped the upper outer quadrant of Linda's right buttock with an alcohol swab. "One, two . . ." *En garde!* In it went, with no flinching by Linda. I pulled out the plunger and looked closely at the chamber. It was clear. In went the plunger for the distance, as I pushed it with one hand and held the syringe steady with the other. I pulled the needle out, then used another swab to wipe away the dot of blood. I felt my forehead get cool as the relief set in. I had done it right, and knew it would be no problem from then on.

After that first night I wasn't nervous at all giving Linda the shots, but I always felt funny about how it was done—coming at her from behind as if conducting a surprise attack. There was also an ironic twist. When I thought I had inserted the needle awkwardly and saw a lot of bleeding afterward, Linda told me it didn't hurt at all. When I thought the needle had gone in and out with a straight and smooth motion, she often said it hurt more than usual. And the short-needle Lupron injections in the thigh, which were easy for me, sometimes caused her more pain than the Pergonal ones.

Meanwhile, Dr. Gold didn't let me remain drug-free. He gave me a prescription for a powerful and expensive antibiotic called Cipro to knock off any bacteria that might be in my semen and that could interfere with fertilization. I got this treatment only because I had had a high count of white blood cells in my samples that could have indicated infection. Luckily, my prescription was covered by insurance, unlike Linda's far more costly drug regimen.

On the August morning we took off for the trip, I was armed with a bottle of Valium, courtesy of Dr. Flexner, and my biofeedback device (already on its second 9-volt battery). My fear of what lay ahead was on simmer. Linda was equipped with an assortment of hypodermic needles (in two sizes), ampules of Pergonal, and an apparent calm that I would have paid any amount of money for.

So our journey entered phase three—from trying to have a child the normal way, to trying to figure out why we couldn't have a child the normal way, to replacing the normal way with an array of artificial baby-making technologies. Linda's body would be manipulated by drugs, her reproductive system turned into an egg hatchery with a high production quota. My contribution of sperm seemed like a tiny part of the success formula.

On the flight I closed my eyes periodically but couldn't sleep. While Linda read next to me, I began thinking we were nuts to be getting our treatment long-distance. We'd have to drive through the infamous LA traffic, shell out dough for hotels and rental cars and restaurant meals. Yet, I also thought a change of scene might have a positive effect. I tried to convince myself that infertility was an East Coast problem, like sleet in winter. No way it could have followed our trail across the Mississippi River, over the Rocky Mountains, across the Mojave Desert.

While driving to the clinic in our rental car the next day, my mind was riveted on my upcoming assignment. This was not just a semen test; they were going to keep my sample on ice as a backup in case something went wrong the day of the IVF, although thawed samples were far less potent than the fresh stuff.

My fears were magnified after we arrived at the clinic. The room where I was to produce the sample was barely bigger than a walk-in closet. I'd expected a VCR with a stack of porno tapes to choose from, but all I had to work with were a few copies of *Hustler* and *Penthouse*. I was surrounded by state-of-the-art medical technology, and they had isolated me in a low-tech pleasure center!

Worst of all, the room was right off a well-trafficked hallway. As I was trying to get my pud to snap to attention, I could hear a couple of doctors talking about local traffic conditions that morning. Linda had offered to join me in there but I'd declined. I knew I was going to sink or swim with my head rather than my glands, that Linda's being there would only wreck my concentration.

As I stormed around my tiny space, I began realizing that, despite everything Linda was going through, I had it a lot rougher. Sure, she had to face some discomfort, but she didn't have to *do* anything. I was the one who had to perform again and again, with narrow windows of opportunity constantly putting the pressure on. She didn't have to have an orgasm to get pregnant, but I did!

After what seemed like hours, I emerged into the hallway with my sample in a plastic cup. I felt as if I'd just come out of a centrifuge at the astronaut tryouts. Sweat was rolling down my cheeks and paranoia was racing through my head.

"How did it go?" asked Linda calmly as I approached her in the waiting room. I asked her if she'd wondered what was taking me so long. She looked at me questioningly. I checked my watch and was shocked to see I'd been in there only twenty minutes.

Despite everything working out, I decided that I'd produce my sample for the IVF itself in our room at the inn. I'd have plenty of space and quiet. And a "Do Not Disturb" sign on the door.

For the next few days, we really didn't have to do much other than show up for brief tests at Dr. Gold's office. The rest of the time we were disguised as tourists. We watched the beautiful people Rollerblade in Venice. I stepped into Humphrey Bogart's footprints at Grauman's Chinese Theatre. We drove up the coast and down the coast. These side trips didn't just take our minds off what was going on; in spite of the drama and the pressure, we were somehow having a great vacation and communicating with each other better than we had in a long time. We seemed to be reclaiming a part of our relationship lost during the relentless quest back east.

A standard part of Dr. Gold's IVF program was a visit to a therapist before the procedure, mainly for advice on how the woman could relax after the embryo transfer—when the fertilized embryos were taken from the incubator and placed in her uterus. It was imperative for the woman to lie absolutely still for two hours.

When we went to see Dr. Holman, we found her instantly likable: chatty in a give-and-take way that put us all on equal footing. She had no trace of the official air of Dr. Flexner, and wore a free-flowing moo-moo with a hippieish look to it. No office or electronic recliners there either; we sat in her plant-filled den.

The session took an unexpected turn early on. Although I was ostensibly there as moral support and to gather tips for helping Linda relax, the attention turned to me when I mentioned my high anxiety over producing a semen specimen.

Dr. Holman recommended a way to defuse my anguish in the days that remained before the IVF: spend fifteen minutes a day purposely imagining the worst-case scenario for my particular anxiety, then walk away from it. It hardly seemed pleasant, but made perfect sense. The principle was simple: if I had already imagined something worse than was possible happening, the actual event would seem almost tame. Then I realized that what she was talking about sounded familiar: I'd been doing the same thing all through the infertility—when I had produced semen samples, undergone surgery, given Linda injections. My problem had been that my imagination had controlled me instead of my controlling it.

Dr. Holman didn't suggest this technique right away. It came after a long discussion about my self-image, confidence, childhood, and other components of my psyche that used up virtually all the time of the session. Linda didn't sit silently through it, either; she continually chimed in with her own observations of me over the years to guide Dr. Holman's probing. By the time the appointment was wrapping up, not one piece of advice had been offered to Linda.

On the drive back to the inn, I apologized to Linda and told her that I could help her hone her relaxation skills with my biofeedback device. She waved me off, telling me not to worry about it, that she'd be fine.

As the car crawled through the dense traffic so far from home and so far from the innocence of our first forays into procreative sex, I came to some disturbing realizations. I no longer knew when Linda was sugarcoating her reaction in order to protect my vulnerable psyche. I also wasn't sure if I could tell the difference between being optimistic and just pretending to be. We were two people who knew each other intimately yet who also now harbored secrets, circling each other on the floor like wrestlers about to attack or dancers about to embrace—I couldn't tell which.

I had become a bundle of explosives, with new fuses continually being lit and extinguished just in time. Linda seemed amazingly serene through everything, but maybe I was missing key signals simply because I didn't want to see them. I knew that I fed off her demeanor in some mysterious way, that my knowing or believing she was calm was a critical part of the combination of biofeedback, therapy, and mind games that kept me intact.

A few more days, or a few weeks, months at the most, and then we could straighten all this out, I told myself. It was what I had been telling myself for years.

My first premeditated anxiety attack would have made an X-rated silent film comedy. I set the countdown on my digital watch at fifteen minutes. Ready, set, go. I saw myself not being able to get an erection. Spilling hot coffee into my sample. Catching my penis in the bathroom door before I could get it up. Getting stuck in an elevator with my sample for hours until all the sperm died. Being tied to my bed and forced to have intercourse with a chambermaid, draining my supply before I could produce my sample. Having a cloud of especially toxic LA smog pass over my groin that leaves me with *The Incredible Shrinking Dick.*

As D day approached, I felt that Dr. Holman's technique and my continued biofeedback had lowered the ceiling of my anxiety enough. The day before the scheduled egg retrieval, I gave Linda a shot of human chorionic gonadotropin (HCG), which replaced her normal surge of a hormone that helped the eggs mature.

I drove Linda to the facility early the next morning. Then I returned to our room and produced my sample with surprising ease, without the help of even one centerfold from the assortment of glossy magazines I had taken out of the clinic. After I returned to the facility—with the car's air-conditioning on high to protect my sample from the summer heat, and a towel covering it to shade it from sunlight—the best swimmers in my sperm sample were captured in a special culture.

Linda had responded well to the Pergonal, producing sixteen eggs for the cycle. We decided to try to fertilize twelve of them with my sperm and four of them with the donor's. The sperm-and-egg mixtures would then be put in an incubator for forty-eight hours.

Tall blond stranger had a perfect day at the plate, fertilizing all of his eggs. My minor leaguers managed to penetrate seven of their twelve. We didn't consider using any of the donor embryos; they were frozen as part of our "account" at the clinic, in case we wanted to use them in the future. So were three of mine. (No one wants to risk quadruplets.)

The embryo transfer was scheduled for the following morning, giving them another twenty-four hours to develop more cells and thus become more viable. But my job wasn't over yet. The night before the embryos checked into Linda's womb, we were supposed to have intercourse. Having sex was thought to improve the conditions for implantation. Through all our briefing and prepping for the IVF, I must have been told this, but I couldn't remember a thing about it. Linda yet again tried to provide an escape route, saying we didn't *have* to do it. But with only about one in five IVF procedures resulting in an actual baby, I wasn't about to alter the formula one iota. After an extralong biofeedback session and extended foreplay, I was able to have my final orgasm in the IVF schedule of events.

Linda seemed a bit tense the next day through breakfast and then at the clinic. I caressed her shoulder as she lay on the table. Dr. Gold came in with a couple of technicians and told us he'd come back in a few minutes with the embryos, which would then be transferred via a thin plastic tube through her cervix and into her uterus.

When he returned with our payload, I stroked Linda's head as Dr. Gold positioned her on the table. I looked forward to witnessing a birth someday, but the unnaturalness of this phase still scared me and I had no desire to watch a tube being inserted into my wife's vagina. I tried to concentrate completely on providing moral and physical support for Linda, and carefully avoided looking at Dr. Gold.

The insertion had to be done quickly, but it seemed as if Dr. Gold was down there with our tentative future for a hell of a long time. Suddenly he leaped back from Linda, and the surgical mask was unable to disguise the look of nervousness on his face. He mumbled some words I couldn't understand, but clearly something had gone wrong. With exceptional difficulty, and with me having to hold Linda in a certain position for what seemed like forever, the procedure was eventually completed.

I couldn't believe that Linda would be pretty much allowed to do whatever she wanted by the next day, but that's what Dr. Gold said. Just no heavy exertion. We became tourists again, spending a night at a bed-and-breakfast in the mountains. Around 3:00 A.M. I got up to go to the bathroom. Out the window was the clearest sky I'd seen in years. As I scanned the blanket of stars that surrounded a full moon, I let myself think that they were shining only on me and that no one else at that moment was looking skyward. I hoped God would show me a shooting star to make a wish on, as a sign that he had heard my prayers. I stayed there for a good half hour waiting, but didn't see one.

None of the embryos placed into Linda became fetuses. All we gained from our West Coast expedition was the knowledge that my low-quality sperm could fertilize. The odds had already been against us, and the difficulty of our procedure in particular had made the odds even worse. It was a blow, but not anywhere near as upsetting as our miscarriage three years earlier. Maybe it was the surprising pleasure of our sight-seeing combined with the low expectation of success that kept my depression from sinking too low. Having a failure back home, despite the lower cost, would have seemed much worse.

That fall we decided to visit Dr. Myers, another highly touted fertility specialist. Entering his domain was like confronting the Wizard of Oz. It was almost dark and almost empty but for a bookcase on one wall and a huge desk where he sat to present his exalted opinions to us. No casual joking around like with Dr. Gold; Dr. Myers spoke almost in a whisper, yet with a resonance that radiated authority and compelled full attention.

Dr. Myers voiced optimism for us due to our two pregnancies, as if we were mere borderline infertile despite our six years–plus in the chase. We asked him if he thought artificial insemination (AI) was a viable option, and he said yes. Dr. Gold had already told us that AI would probably be a waste of time for us, but we were eager for something less involved than IVF. And Dr. Myers had such an air of brilliance around him that I felt his support of AI made it an excellent option.

We felt strangely confident after leaving his office. I would still have to produce a sample on-site, but I wasn't even worried about it. Dr. Myers also had a game plan for helping us avoid miscarriage if we did get pregnant. A blood test revealed that Linda had a high level of antinuclear antibodies, which indicated the possibility of an autoimmune reaction triggered by her pregnancy that caused her to miscarry. Disturbing as this news was, it was also gratifying to hear something new and potentially meaningful revealed to us about our situation. Especially since there were treatments to protect against this problem.

A few weeks later we were back in Dr. Myers's office. I produced my sample with ease in a tiny room and handed it over. Once the pipette containing the ammo was in position through Linda's cervix, the technician asked me to squeeze the rubber bulb that delivered my sperm to the target; me at the controls of my surrogate member. After I squeezed it, she pulled out the pipette and Linda had to lie still for a few minutes. That was it.

As we drove home I felt certain that the procedure had worked. No complicated out-of-body sperm-and-egg rendezvous where so much could go wrong. No problems getting through Linda's cervix. In a few months, when Linda's belly was out to here, we'd laugh about all the histrionics we went through, when a simple procedure barely one step removed from the old in-out could have done the job all along.

Two failed attempts later, I was not so confident. Dr. Gold had probably been right about AI. Maybe some medical guru or holistic shaman had a solution to our problem, but I didn't know how to find him or if I could summon enough energy to begin the search. The fact was, there was probably no end to the medical treatments available to us. New technologies for combating infertility were being developed all the time; the only things stopping us from trying them all were our decreasing finances and Linda's increasing age.

She was about to turn thirty-seven. I'd turn forty a month after that. And I knew that the wish echoing in my head as I tried to extinguish the candles crowding my cake, the same wish I'd made for the last six years, would be as ephemeral as my breath snuffing the flames.

# Chapter 9

# Gold Rush

It was the year of the Rodney King riots and the Martin Luther King Day earthquake and the mud slides. Dr. Gold had been back in Los Angeles for two years and was wondering whether God was trying to give him a hint. On the phone I asked him about the practice, about how his wife and sons were doing. He made fun of New York, I made fun of California. Sparring before the main event: talk of in vitro.

"We're not movie stars," I said. "We don't jet across the country to have exotic procedures performed." The truth was, I knew I wouldn't go through with it unless Ed and I did just that. The other possibility was the IVF star of the era, the Cornell University Medical Center in Manhattan. But it had a two-year waiting list. And it didn't have Dr. Gold—not the biggest celebrity among fertility doctors, but certainly the one who would give us the most personal attention, a factor I did not discount in assessing our chances for pregnancy.

He and I had spoken lots of times since he moved away, and I was still drawn to him as a doctor and as a person. He was vulnerable and accessible beneath the medical exterior, and

I couldn't help feeling pulled toward him. He and a nurse at his California clinic, Karen, had already spoken to us about the logistics of doing this complicated procedure long-distance; we wouldn't be the first Gold groupies to go through it. We'd need to be in LA for about a week. All the preliminary and follow-up work could be done in conjunction with a clinic back east. But I had ticked off Dr. Gold's colleague in our local clinic by talking to one of the nurses there about that possibility. Dr. Richards, who had occasionally seen me during the Zoladex treatment and seemed a nice enough fellow, was now furious that I wasn't having the lucrative IVF procedure done with him. He actually called me at work—the first time I ever spoke with him outside the clinic—in order to make me feel bad about it. Then said: "I remember you, from filling out all those Zoladex forms. You're like JFK to me."

What a strange man, I thought. What did he mean? Mine sounded like a famous historical name because of all the documents of a pharmaceutical trial? Or my name had gotten jumbled up with his schoolboy memorization of names and facts? Or did he think he was being charming and funny, getting in good with me?

He caught me off guard. How could I explain to him why I would rather fly out to Los Angeles to have a doctor I trusted and liked perform the in vitro procedure than just have it done by him thirty-five minutes from my house? It was none of his business, really, but I couldn't react fast enough to his undeserved indignation.

I told all this to Dr. Gold on the phone. It was one of those startlingly perfect June days, and Ed and I were about to play hooky and take a long drive in the country. I had just run back into the house for my sunglasses when Dr. Gold returned my call.

"I don't think of you as JFK," he said in response. "I think of you as a beautiful woman with dark hair and a nice husband, and I'd like to help you."

I didn't hear much of what he said after that, or much of what anyone said in the next few days. He thought I was beautiful. *Beautiful.* My infatuation had just been given permission to crank itself way up. It flashed across my mind that he, too, was just vying for a chance to do a lucrative procedure, but he was my friend. I trusted him. By the time I hung up the phone, I knew I would be able to go through with the in vitro.

On our drive that day, every song that came on the radio or that we played on a tape seemed to be about the possibility of David Gold and me being together. He was the brother, the savior, the lover I never had. I was treading dangerously close to the place where infatuation became something more. For now, I just wanted to give Dr. Gold the chance to dazzle us with his fancy procedure. And to give Ed and me a chance that might make all the difference (though we knew that, at best, that chance was only 20 percent). It would be ridiculous, just ridiculous, to say that I underwent in vitro fertilization just so I could see Dr. Gold again, but one way or another I wanted to hear him whisper to me those three little words: "You're pregnant, Linda."

When I announced to Ed that weekend, after months of waffling, that, yes, I'd be willing to undergo IVF, he just stood in the kitchen and stared at me with a stone face. I'd felt I was coming through with a magnanimous sacrifice. Baffled by his glumness, I exploded in confusion and forced him to explain why he was reacting as if I had just told him I'd leave him unless we moved back to Manhattan and remained childless.

He was grappling with quite a different scenario. If I was letting myself drift into a fantasy romance with a very married physician three thousand miles away, Ed was watching helplessly as a shark cage of performance anxiety was lowered onto him. He was terrified of having to produce a sperm sample on demand and had already, I could see, been thinking way too much about it. And here I'd thought that getting thrice-daily injections for six weeks and undergoing two medical procedures made the IVF about *me*.

I sympathized with him, I really did, but he was taking a nervousness that any man might have under such circumstances and constructing of it a monster of obsession. Soon we'd have packages of hypodermics and thousands of dollars' worth of ovary-enhancing drugs in the house. My body would be run by hormones made from the urine of menopausal nuns (don't ask: that's where they came from then). But the specter of Ed trying to jerk off in a room somewhere in a West Coast doctor's office was what was going to drive the engine of this process.

We had created an entity that would allow us to pursue in vitro. Not that of a devoted couple making the difficult decision to move on to a high-tech, fairly desperate level of medical onslaught. But a husband forcing himself to confront an obsessional fear in order to pursue an obsessional goal. And a wife pretending to live out the soap opera plot of the attentive, adorable doctor and his ailing patient—sick enough to require his continual care, but not so sick that she doesn't appear before him in full makeup, her dark hair flowing across the white pillowcase of her hospital bed.

Two months later, after the excruciation of following the complicated instructions long-distance, after the injections and tests had begun, we packed a suitcase and all that other baggage and got on a plane. We were headed to La-La Land to make a baby.

The thing about LA is that it is 1954 there. I expected sunniness and glamour, Disney and surfers. I did not expect to encounter likenesses of Marilyn Monroe and James Dean and to see fifties-style diners at every turn.

I am, let us say, not a confident driver, so Ed handled the rental car. The freeway is no place for amateurs. If I had tried to drive along it, with my jerky lane changes and inability to tell how much room I had, my panicky misjudgings—"Can I go? Can I go?"—I'd be like the tourists and suburbanites who flood Manhattan sidewalks at Christmastime. They stop dead in the throng along Fifth Avenue to lean down into a stroller or unfurl a map. They haven't learned the rhythm necessary to peaceful coexistence on those crowded streets. They have no business being there; they could cause a serious accident. When it's done right—the speeding up and slowing down, the veering toward and away from one's fellow travelers—it's a stupendous connection, exciting and life-affirming as foreplay.

Ed drove and drove around the sprawl of LA. In between being monitored at the clinic, we took in the sights. (From Universal Studios, I checked in with Dr. Gold by phone. It was a miserably hot day, an uncharacteristic heat wave. "I'm in the third circle of hell," I told him. "Stay hydrated!" he ordered. Somehow it seemed the sexiest thing anyone had ever said to me.) I emphatically did *not* want to see Disneyland, imagining it as a daunting, impossibly commercial place for kids.

We were staying at a pretty inn not far from Dr. Gold's office. The evening we arrived, we settled in our room and walked over to its restaurant for dinner. I felt a pull, knowing my doctor was minutes away. I hadn't seen him since Ed and I had taken him out for a farewell dinner two years before. He normally didn't allow patients to take him out as a thank-you after getting them pregnant, but he had cheerily considered my invitation and decided it would be proper for a couple considering in vitro to discuss it with him over dinner.

The dynamics of the three of us were unbalanced. The service was slow. Out in public, fully dressed, I wasn't able to slip into the clinic persona I had perfected with my doctor. I wasn't spunky. I didn't make him laugh. The evening was uncomfortable, though he seemed his usual buoyant self.

Outside in the parking lot, I tried to say good-bye to this man who had taken on a role in my life I did not want to relinquish. I handed him a greeting card I had laboriously written out by way of good-bye. I had been reading Robertson Davies at the time and my head was filled with his rhythms. I tried to sound profound and literary, tried to let my doctor read between the proper lines to let him know I was mad for him. But more: that I liked him, that I was grateful for his decency and kindness through what could have been nothing more than a series of humiliating showdowns. I couldn't bring myself to tell him in the card that I was devastated by his departure, but I did tell him that I would remember him and miss him.

He shook hands with Ed, then turned to me. I felt we were exactly the same height, looking straight into each other's faces.

It was a nice new feeling, after years of arcing up to meet my husband's face, seven inches over mine. Dr. Gold turned to Ed and asked in a nervous whisper, "Can I kiss her?" When Ed nodded, my doctor gave me an affectionate peck on the cheek, and we hugged. I knew I was losing something important and irretrievable, something that would leave a sizable hole in my life, something I would later think I hadn't appreciated enough at the time. Committed medical help, sure, but something much more. It was getting late. We had kept him too long from his wife. We headed off in separate directions for our cars, and he was gone.

Now, walking through the doors of this burnished restaurant in LA, I was overcome with a sudden sensation of David Gold. It flooded through me like a visit from a ghost, like an electric current of certainty, as my eyes fell on an enormous vase of fresh flowers. Ed and I were led through the back doors and out onto the patio. Minutes later, while we examined menus and enjoyed the soothing California air, my eyes were summoned up and I spotted the figure of my doctor crisscrossing the lawn outside the gated dining area, trying to find his way in.

Just as he had when he greeted Dr. Gold at the farewell dinner back east, Ed now placed his tall, broad-shouldered silhouette between me and my doctor, completely obscuring my view of him. The marital screen was suddenly lifted, and there he was, next to me. "I *knew* I'd find you here," Dr. Gold said, giving me a friendly hug. We hadn't expected to see him until the next morning in his office, but he'd spontaneously decided to stop by after work. When we invited him to join us for dinner, he said he'd love to, but couldn't. He just sat at our table for a few minutes, visiting, asking questions, going over with us again what to expect in the coming days.

"I'm dying to test your sperm," he said to Ed—then immediately surveyed the surrounding tables with a grimace, fearful of what that line might sound like out of context. He seemed wound up, excited. It was a great ego boost, I guess, to have a patient travel three thousand miles to you for treatment. And I needed to think, too, that he was happy to see me. I stared greedily at his familiar hands with the jagged wedding band (his wife wore the interlocking piece), at his mustache and dark, eager eyes. I sat between him and Ed, the two men who would get me through this $8,000 procedure.

When we got back to our room, there was a voice-mail message from Dr. Gold welcoming us to LA. I knew then that at the precise moment he was making that call, before leaving his office on a hunch that he would find us, I was feeling the rush of his presence in the restaurant. I don't buy into that stuff, really—although I come from a family who reads tea leaves and pays psychics to tell them their future—but it happened, more than once, when it came to Dr. Gold.

The next morning Ed and I showed up at his office for an ultrasound. From what I had been reading in preparation for the IVF, I had a faint worry at the back of my mind. "Do you think Pergonal can increase a woman's risk of getting ovarian cancer?" I asked Dr. Gold. "You're worrying about that *now*?" he responded with incredulity. He didn't answer my question, though. What the hell was I doing?

Ed and I each put half the cost of the procedure on our Visa cards. For some reason, the receptionist had trouble processing the charge, and as we stood there with the credit card machine between us and the medical personnel it occurred to me that we were involved in something absurd. Between the cost of the drugs, the unreimbursable procedure, and the trip to California, Ed and I had rung up a five-figure bill. We'd be paying it off until Junior learned how to ride a bike.

Medically, I responded very well. I never got used to Ed coming after me with a hypodermic, though. Some shots were nearly painless, others were tough to take. Still, I think I'd rather have been the recipient than the giver. "No matter how badly he handles the injections," one of the nurses had advised me, "tell him it was great." "Hmm. Just like sex, huh?" I responded, but no one laughed. I told Ed when it was great (which wasn't too many times), and I told him when it hurt. The bruises would have given me away anyway.

My obedient ovaries, in response to the expensive pharmaceuticals, produced sixteen eggs that month. I was a great candidate. My uterine lining had thickened to a hospitable pillow; the medications were having no bad side effects. I'd read through all my newsletters from Resolve (a national organization for infertiles) to bring questions and problems to mind that I wouldn't have thought of on my own. I knew that an injection of HCG would be administered when the eggs were ready to be "retrieved," which would be done under light general anesthesia by Dr. Gold, who would aspirate them out of my ovaries vaginally through a thin needle. Two days later, after they'd mixed with Ed's sperm and formed healthy "pre-embryos" that would bubble up as they divided in a petri dish, the all-important embryo transfer into my uterus would take place.

Now, this was supposed to be the easy part. All you had to do was let the doctor thread a catheter up your vagina and shoot in the embryos, then lie perfectly still for two hours hoping the living cells would attach themselves to the wall of your uterus. His anxiety notwithstanding, Ed not only managed to supply sperm on demand but to fertilize seven of his twelve eggs; the other four of the sixteen I'd produced were paired up with a donor—Ed's panicky backup in case he couldn't perform on cue. I'm stunned now to think that I'd agreed to accept embryos made from a stranger's sperm—the bizarre cold-blooded intimacy of it, the hybrid child who might be made from it. When it came to the infertility, after a while I just followed the script Ed handed me. This was his show.

In the end, we used only four of Ed's embryos (to lessen the risk of multiple births) and none of the donor's. I had been shown the room where the embryo transfers took place, with two tables specially built for the procedure. Depending on which way your uterus tipped, you would lie on your back or your stomach for the procedure, calling on gravity to help. Here's how it played out on that sunny morning.

I woke up nervous. The mirrored closets and good lighting in our room made it seem I was seeing myself clearly for the first time. "Don't tank up on coffee," Dr. Gold had advised, "or you'll have to pee." I ate a light breakfast with Ed. I was distracted, and couldn't even wait for him to finish. I went back to our room alone to fuss and pace.

When we got to Dr. Gold's office I told him I felt nervous. I'd been calm before all those surgeries, even the egg retrieval two days prior. "What, you don't want to have a baby?" he said, smiling. Did I? Or was I just having a premonition of the tragicomedy of errors that was about to unfold?

I was allowed to keep on the loose oversized white shirt I was wearing. All I'd have to do was strip from the waist down and climb aboard the embryo-transfer table. Dr. Gold gave me a quickie pelvic exam on the spot and determined that I'd need to be lying on my stomach for the procedure.

The table was a marvel of in vitro technology. It bent in the middle, was adjustable from seemingly all directions. So how come it wouldn't accommodate me? My butt, I could see with dismay, was going to form the apex of an upside-down V, but something was very, very wrong with my top half. No matter how the table was adjusted, I slid off. Stumped, the nurses and technicians planted Ed in front of me and instructed him to buttress me by pushing against my elbows. I couldn't help but push back with all my might. How the hell was I supposed to relax during this critical procedure with every muscle in my body at full attention? I was on a table made for women having in vitro, but it was so antithetical to my proportions and my anatomy that it might as well have been a machine to extract semen from a bull.

Apparently I was a freak the likes of which they had never seen. Was it my height? ("A tall drink of water," Dr. Gold said when one of the nurses commented on my size.) Some odd distribution of weight? As I contorted myself into more and more unnatural positions, I felt as if I were on some strange amusement park ride. "And I said I wasn't going to Disneyland!" I announced to the group around me.

By the time we finagled a workable position, my attention was diverted away from the table and the likelihood of the procedure's success and toward just one thing: in moments I would be mooning a roomful of doctors and nurses under unforgiving hospital lights. Ed assured me that the paper drape over my rump would remain during the procedure, but Dr. Gold indifferently explained otherwise. When we seemed ready, he instructed the technicians to bring in the embryos, which were stored in a special culture medium in an incubator, outside of which they could remain for only three minutes before their viability would be compromised. I was facing away from everybody and everything, but after a few quiet moments I became acutely aware that there was a problem. Dr. Gold was having difficulty, major difficulty, getting the catheter through my cervix.

When he sent the technicians to put our embryos back in the incubator, I knew we were in trouble. What the hell was wrong with me? First I couldn't even fit on a table designed for women undergoing this procedure, then my cervix decided to close up shop at its starring moment. I remembered that Dr. Gold had had the same difficulty two years before, when he'd tried to do an endometrial biopsy, and cursed myself for not remembering to remind him of it.

Ed and I had both noticed how California life had slowed down Dr. Gold. He didn't move with the same jerky, fast motions. He no longer talked at a New York clip. But later Ed would tell me that Dr. Gold leaped back from the in vitro table when he came across the impenetrable cervix. And Dr. Gold himself would tell me he had been shaking. Of all embryo transfers, mine! The patient he was so fond of, one of the ones who had come all the way from New York. It was as if we had decided to have an affair, and he just couldn't get it up.

I lay on the table staring at a blank wall while my doctor, my husband, and several technicians hovered, whispering, shuffling. The embryos were brought back in. Dr. Gold tried again. By now, I was beginning to feel very sore and put upon. My cervix was bleeding from the assault, I'd later learn. Eventually they called a halt. This Hollywood crew was on break. They went back to their trailers, poured coffee. I sat up, wrapped a drape around my bottom half, walked around. Dr. Gold chatted nervously. I was now calm as could be. I was just concerned because I knew another woman was scheduled for an embryo transfer after mine; she and her husband had to wait because of my cervical drama.

Dr. Gold's boss, the head of a whole string of fertility clinics, happened to be visiting that day. He was a large, flamboyant man. Dr. Gold explained to him the trouble he'd been having, and this new doctor, who'd seen his share of difficult embryo transfers, offered to step in. The mood in the room lightened. I seem to remember a promotional videotape for the clinics being played for a few minutes at some point, and much lighthearted banter. They were stalling. I felt like saying, "I'm ready for my close-up."

After a long while the replacement doctor got down to business. "Let's make you a mama!" he shouted, and we all took up our positions again. It took some doing—I'd say Take 4 or 5, counting Dr. Gold's attempts—but he managed to complete the transfer, and suddenly there was no one in the room but Ed and me. The table was leveled so that I could lie comfortably. My butt was mercifully covered. ("Is a pink blanket okay?" a nurse asked, smiling. "In case it influences the sex of the baby?") For two hours I lay there, my cervix burning from the trauma, feeling as if I'd die if I didn't get to a bathroom. We followed the instructions as if they still applied. But I think both

Ed and I knew that it would take more than the usual miracle for this IVF to succeed.

So we weren't that hurt or surprised when we found out it hadn't. The worst part was having to call on the services of an old medical school buddy of Dr. Gold's for the results after we got home. He was an obstetrician in an upscale town. Someone in his office had drawn blood, and when I kept calling to find out whether I was pregnant, the receptionist couldn't understand my urgency. When she finally told me the results were negative, she said, "Well, just try again this month, honey." Yeah. Thanks for the advice.

After I hung up the phone, I saw that day's *Times* on the kitchen table. On the front page was a picture of a Somali child with pencil-thin limbs and a beautiful face drawn taut and wasted from starvation. It was so hard not to lose perspective. For the three years that remained of our infertility struggle, every time I felt myself leaning toward self-pity, the "Why me?" of the moderately stricken middle class, I brought to mind the photograph of that child and reminded myself that our infertility was a wrenching personal problem but it was not a tragedy.

When it was all over, and I had no reason to see Dr. Gold anymore, when he finally told me I could call him by his first name, we drifted out of touch but I'd always send a card around the holidays. I could not let go of the force he had been in my life for five years. After receiving one of my cards, he wrote back a short note that elated me more than it had any right to. "I miss you," he'd written at the end in his boyish script, then signed it, "Fondly (*fondly!*), David." No intimation of ardor or lust. Something much better: the simple declaration that he wished our paths could still cross. He'd given me the gift I always crave: he'd known me well.

Was I in love with him? No, I don't think so. I may have been in love with the attention he paid, with his kindness and humor, with his undoctorly demeanor, with the way he made me feel through something that was meant to be an ordeal. It was hell, but it wasn't *only* hell. And I knew I had David Gold to thank for that.

An obligation had been met, I felt. When you've gotten this far in infertility treatment, some of us believe, you've got to take your chances with IVF. If it doesn't work, well, at least you tried.

Ed and I coasted through the next few months, drifting inevitably toward the next treatment. In my holiday card to Dr. Gold at the end of the year, I wrote jauntily, stupidly, "I believe you have something of ours out there that we may come out to claim." This was a reference to the three unused embryos (made with Ed's sperm), which had been frozen for possible use in a future IVF cycle. The next time I spoke to Dr. Gold on the phone, he had a different procedure in mind.

Rather than de-ice those potentially life-forming treasures, a process that decreases the already extremely low chance of successful pregnancy, he wanted us to try GIFT—for gamete intra-fallopian transfer. This variation on plain old in vitro involves a laparoscopy and allows egg and sperm to unite in the fallopian tube (bypassing my ungracious cervix) rather than in a petri dish. The new embryo can then tumble down to the uterus at its own natural pace. What's more,

Dr. Gold pointed out, since I'd be an endometriosis patient having a laparoscopy, our insurance would cover the surgical part of the procedure.

Why not? The stakes were getting higher, but we were still in the game. The long night of gambling was drawing to a close, though, both Ed and I realized, so we hedged our bets. There was no way we were going to leave our own biological embryos unused; some high-tech procedure or other was going to be tried at some point. But we had also attended an adoption conference, and were starting to get an idea of the mammoth undertaking of private adoption. (The alternatives were foreign adoption, which didn't feel right for us, and agency adoption, which takes years and years and often has age cutoffs we would never make.) Psychologically and logistically, it would be best to make preparations for that now.

Between the acts—between August 1992, when we underwent IVF, and April 1993, when we'd fly out to LA again for GIFT—I'd spoken to a friend who'd gotten pregnant with another fertility specialist. Dr. Gold was gone and Dr. Richards would have made me feel uncomfortable at our old clinic—not to mention that once or twice when I went there after Dr. Gold's departure, I'd had an hour-and-a-half wait, with no explanation. It wasn't the same place. So Ed and I made an appointment with the competition. It felt strange, disloyal, but maybe there was something he could add to the mix.

We told Dr. Myers that we'd undergone one in vitro and would probably eventually do GIFT, but that we knew there were some low-tech options we had bypassed. It was of "spectacular importance," he told us, that we had gotten pregnant twice on our own. With this new doctor, we underwent two predictably unsuccessful attempts at artificial insemination, for which poor Ed once again had to perform on command. And something new showed up in a blood test. I had an elevated level of ANA, antinuclear antibodies, which can interfere with the embryo's implantation and lead to miscarriage. Usually this was treated with heparin, but the cutting-edge approach was intravenous immunoglobulin. My insurance would cover it, but it was an experimental treatment.

I was always glad to have some new problem identified. It meant that it might be remedied and that everything might suddenly work. We'd been in fertility treatment for six years, though. What I didn't know but would read about later is that the longer you're in treatment, the less likely you are to have a biological child. When years and years pass, it's a good indication that both husband and wife have a medical problem, making it less likely that they'll get there, either on their own or with help.

I didn't understand any of that yet. I understood that this new doctor, with his skylight office and his distant manner, held out a new hope. We grabbed on.

I am lying on a fake leather recliner with my arm in a specially designed rest. A tube leads from a rack on which is hung a plastic bag of whitish liquid that flows through it and into my arm. Our second and last attempt at high-tech intervention looms a few months in the future. As extra insurance, I am being transfused with gamma globulin—a component of blood plasma containing antibodies against certain microorganisms, used to treat measles, hepatitis, and polio—in an effort to bring my

ANA level back to normal. I am in a blood center on the first floor of a local hospital.

I share the large room with people who are here for other reasons. A beautiful young woman wearing a turban leans forward in her seat to have chemicals poured through a hole near her collarbone. A bald young boy with a brain tumor is waiting for his platelets to arrive, and the nurses gather around to entertain him and his mother during the delay. Some of the room's inhabitants are hospital inmates, thin apparitions shuffling around in bathrobes and slippers, wheeling their metal poles around with them. Only I know that I am the one patient here not in dire health, crashing the cancer ward.

The whole of the infertility treatment, I now see, has been a safe rehearsal for that possible time when I will be treated for a life-threatening disease. A dress rehearsal, a death rehearsal. Nothing is degenerating or debilitating me, but I've been put through the paces of someone with a terminal illness. All the pieces are in place: the doctors, the hospitals, the failed surgical procedures, the heartbreaking news to the families.

The infusion takes a while. Patients come and go, some here just to make appointments. The nurses banter constantly, hilariously, but only to one another. A TV set blares inanely: *Truth or Consequences, Rush Limbaugh, Family Feud.* They love it, the nurses, and heatedly debate the merits of game shows versus talk shows. Something reminds one of them of the luscious peaches her aunt ships from Georgia every year. Which jogs the memory of another, who tells a story of coming across wild blackberry bushes in Maine. On vacation, she and her family once gathered a basket of berries and, without a recipe, baked them into a pie. "What a pie!" she said. "I don't know if it was because we picked the berries ourselves, or some special thing we did when we made it, but, I'm telling you, you never tasted anything so delicious. So, of course, we never tried to make it again."

At first I thought her odd. If it was so wonderful, why not try to duplicate it, again and again? Then I decided it was a mature stance, maybe even a common one. Maybe Ed's and my trouble was that we went too far in the other direction. We would have tried to make that pie again forty times, each time agreeing it wasn't as good as the first.

We just won't take no for an answer. Ed was testing his obsession with fatherhood to see how far it would take him. I was traveling along on the crest of some nameless wave. Nobody was going to tell us when to stop. The medical community gave us no reason to. There would always be another procedure, a new drug, a slim chance. And we didn't have the wherewithal to stop this ourselves. Worse, we had something in us that wanted things too strongly. Desperate, we sought them, and, desperately, we lost.

I once heard a story about a family who drove cross-country on vacation with their dog, a beagle who kept its head out the window nearly the whole way. By the time they got to California, the dog was blind. It's not always worth it to look into what you might be missing.

GIFT is going to be the end of the line medically, Ed and I agree going in, so we pull out all the stops: gamma globulin, chiropractic, acupuncture. It requires the same injections as the IVF did to shut down my natural cycle (with the exception of the Lupron injection, now replaced by a nasal spray), but this time we go through it like the pros we are. Ed's needles are swift and clinical. To defray the enormous expense of the Pergonal, I mail my prescription to a pen pal I'd been corresponding with in France since seventh grade. Each ampule costs only $6 there, compared with $50 in the U.S. She dutifully procures the multiple boxes of ampules and wraps them up like a professional packer, but I have to make several transatlantic phone calls in my rusty French to try to track down the package. It arrives the day before the protocol demands that we start taking them.

We visited Ed's family near Phoenix first, then drove to California from there. There was a moment in Utah when Ed pulled over to the side of the road to explore a small cave in the vast, dramatic landscape, while I stayed behind. The light was exceptional and I detected in the vanity mirror a growth of beard under my chin, from all the hormones I'd been taking. I fished a pair of tweezers out of my handbag. And that was the picture of my marriage at that point: Ed spelunking in a dark, remote cave while I took advantage of the natural light to pluck out a dense row of unnatural hairs. There was nobody else, anywhere, to be seen.

I have only impressionistic memories of that second trip to LA. The deep pleasure of seeing Dr. Gold again. Having dinner in a restaurant with him and his wife, feeling stupefied and unattuned in her presence. ("You're shy," he'd say the next day as I sat in his office, surprised at this correct news that his gregarious wife must have given him about me.) Asking to see him on the morning of the laparoscopy, but being put under before I am given the chance. Feeling self-pity when the anesthetist warns me that the fluid he's injecting is going to sting, and then indeed feeling the burn work its way up my arms. Having post-op trouble with the anesthesia again, throwing up in a wheelchair in the empty conference room where I'd been parked. The more serious nurse, whom I remember from the IVF and whose last day at the clinic this is, bickering with a busty, flighty new nurse she is afraid won't succeed without her direction ("Can't you see that this patient is not coming out of the anesthesia properly? She's vomiting and her blood pressure is low. She needs a shot of ephedrine"). Dr. Gold telling me afterward that he "can't imagine that this won't work," so perfectly did everything go this time. Chastising him for using such language to someone in my position, and telling him that, before putting his business card into my wallet, I cut off the graphic, the one showing a pair of hands with an infant inside. Going up to the hotel room after Ed produced his sample there—alone, of course, just him and the girlie magazines the clinic had given him—curious but mortified that my child might come to be as a result of those slutty images of vacant-looking blondes. Being shut up in a hotel room after the surgery, watching bad pay-per-view movies and tending to my incision. (Unlike the freedom I enjoyed after in vitro, recuperation after the surgery of GIFT precluded tourism.) Meeting Dr. Gold for coffee on the Saturday before we leave, thanking him, resisting the urge to put my hand on his knee as we sit together, being joined at our outdoor table by a chatty woman, a stranger coming between me and my doctor in our final moments together: *Brief Encounter* without the encounter.

We've got a few days' wait for the pregnancy test after we get home. Ed and I drive out to Long Island for my nephew

Justin's First Communion. Kneeling in the church, I am overcome by the beauty of these second-graders in their pure white dresses and suits, their hands pressed together in supplication, the girls' clean, shiny hair tied up in ribbons and half-covered by veils, the boys with the faces of angels, all of their perfect little bodies in unison before God. They are holy creatures here, though no doubt holy terrors at home. Yes, I think I would like one of these. Please let me be pregnant with one now, I say to God, blinking back tears.

The Catholic church I attended as a child had tiered rows of candles in bumpy red glass holders near the doors. The tradition is to take a long match to one of the votives to make a prayer and then leave some money in a tin box for each candle you light. I want my prayer to be official, but this modern church has no flames, just electric red candles that are activated by a switch. "Who do we give the offering to?" I ask Ed. "The Long Island Lighting Company?"

Well, the prayer must have found its way to God, because it was answered.

We're thrilled but cautious. Third time's the charm! My parents have been visiting from Florida for Justin's Communion, and I decide to let them in on it, partly because my father had walked in on Ed giving me a progesterone shot in the butt a week before and I figure I owe him an explanation. I've come down with a gut-busting cough, though, and can't take any medication for it. I am finally in a position to tell my parents to expect a grandchild from me, but I literally can't do it. I strain to tell them that I'm pregnant—no, only that "the pregnancy test was positive"—through severe laryngitis, taunting them with every other syllable until they piece together the wonderful news.

We need to find professionals to finish out the GIFT protocol. (When I call Dr. Gold's office, I tell Karen the good news, then he gets on the phone and says, "Is this the one who got knocked up?") First, we need an ultrasound to rule out ectopic pregnancy and locate the embryonic sac safely within the womb. We're boycotting Dr. Gold's old office because of the drop-off in patient care, and the renegade doctor who took us through artificial insemination doesn't do ultrasounds in his office. But he gives us the name of a radiologist who does.

I still can't go to a new doctor's office without feeling a longing for Dr. Gold; he's spoiled me for any other medical person. I don't like this tall, white-haired radiologist. He's curt. He's flip. He tries to make conversation, but it's grating. He doesn't have the more accurate vaginal ultrasound that Dr. Gold always used for the delicate, specialized situation of an infertility patient, but a plain old abdominal one. We situate ourselves for him, explain our embattled history. We are six weeks' pregnant, and he says we may or may not be able to see the sac on the ultrasound screen. Moments later we do see it, and he takes a measurement.

"It's too small," he says abruptly, not looking at us. "No, this is too small for six weeks. This is the size of a five-week sac."

Ed and I hardly have time to register alarm or sorrow. The wiry radiologist keeps up a running commentary so hurtful and so misinformed that I won't feel enraged and vindictive until much later in the day.

"At least you know you can get pregnant," he says. "But you used Pergonal, right? That can make the pregnancy progress more slowly." *What?* "And, you know, just being pregnant, even if you miscarry, will cure your endometriosis." Where did this guy come up with this stuff? How dare he do this to us? This quiet couple beginning to mourn once again. This nice young man and woman just here for an image of their embryo because the gonzo fertility doctor who performed the high-tech procedure to get them pregnant is a day's flight away.

"Let me check your ovaries to see whether you hyperstimulated from the Pergonal." Huh? That's a rare complication that I would have known about weeks ago and been hospitalized for.

We drive home in frozen silence and give Dr. Gold's office a call. Now I am mad that this has happened to us, and I inappropriately release my anger to my doctor. "This *idiot,* this man, actually said that pregnancy *cures* endometriosis! First he said he wasn't sure he would even *see* the embryonic sac, then he said for sure it wasn't big enough—and from just an abdominal ultrasound!"

Dr. Gold let me rant, sympathized with me about having to see this awful doctor, then explained that there is an accuracy of plus or minus five days to these measurements, an estimate made even shakier by the use of an abdominal ultrasound. A second ultrasound in two weeks, when a heartbeat should be able to be picked up, would give us a better indication of where we stood.

I wanted my doctor here through this. Was he holding anything back? What would he have said to us if he had given me the ultrasound himself? Would he have said it was too early to tell? Would he have comforted us and gently prepared us for bad news? I wanted to hug him, to cry on him, to have him see me through this, here, now.

But he was in California now. In California with his wife and his two children and his *new* beautiful patients with their dark hair and their nice husbands.

We called on Dr. Chang. I remembered her saying she could "help keep it cooking" if we got pregnant again. She looked at my back and said immediately, "Mmm, yes, pregnant." Then she touched my lower abdomen, pronouncing it "perfect." She took my pulse, squeezed my nipples, and looked at my tongue, hair, head, ankles, and calves. "Don't tell anybody yet," she said, "but I think it's a boy."

The creepy radiologist would eat his words. This sweet wizard of a woman didn't even charge me for the visit—"a gift for the baby," she said.

During the long subway ride back to Manhattan for the commuter train home, a button popped off the waistband of my skirt. I was pregnant! My clothes were too small. I felt the terrible pleasure of Dr. Chang's words and blessing. It was time to find an obstetrician.

We make an appointment with Dr. D'Angelo, a round, talkative OB who listens raptly to our tale. Except for the visit with the midwife four years earlier, this is the first time we have been released into the mainstream world of baby doctors. He can't believe what we have been through. We are an anomaly, a high-risk pregnancy if ever he has seen one. He whips out a paper wheel designed to calculate a baby's due date. We'd never allowed ourselves this luxury with the other two pregnancies. "You've probably already looked this up, right?" Wrong. He wheels it around and announces: January 12.

We are due for the next ultrasound, but he doesn't have the machinery in his office, either. I had asked ahead of time and been told I could have one done there—but now I learn that it's downstairs in radiology and requires a separate appointment. They're closed for the day. All he can do today is give me a pelvic. Feeling the soft, slightly enlarged uterus, he announces with glee, "You're pregnant as hell!"

The next day we show up downstairs for an ultrasound. This time they at least have the vaginal kind, but the technician wants me to guide the wand into my vagina myself. I find it is a tricky business. Dr. Gold had always glided it in effortlessly. For me, it's a dildo I'm having trouble manipulating. The lubricating gel . . . the insertion . . . it's not far enough in. I feel like a high school girl in the backseat of her boyfriend's car.

She discreetly returns and begins swinging it back and forth to locate the embryo. She's very young. She's not a doctor. She adjusts the controls on the screen, grows quiet after I tell her our history. "Sometimes, I don't know, the man upstairs . . . ," she says. At first I think she is referring to Dr. D'Angelo, then I realize it's a cosmic complaint.

We're looking for a heartbeat. We're not finding it yet. "Does the sac look small to you for eight weeks?" I ask. She can't say for sure yet, she responds. She won't take her eyes off the screen. "Can you find a heartbeat yet?" The questions from Ed and me float up to her in softer and softer tones. We can see the image of our baby. It looks like every picture of every embryo I've ever seen. She's trying to zero in on it to examine it. It's a computer game or graphics job. She needs to stop and consult with someone. The ultrasound wand is removed. A familiar dread begins to rise in me. Always, I realize, I am braced for bad news. I am braced for it now. I have been through this before. I can handle it.

My husband's face reveals a different message, an utter sadness I need to protect him from. I tell him I'd rather he leave the room, that it's going to take a long time and I'm not comfortable with him there. I insist. I don't want him to remember the image of his baby who has no heartbeat. Ed leaves reluctantly, silently, for the waiting room, and the technician returns with a doctor I don't know. I put the wand back in place. The image grows larger, then larger still. It is not alive. The young technician has not come across this before. If I were in Dr. Gold's office, I would be expected to collapse in tears. But here I'm the one in control. I need to show the way to these neophytes.

I dress and collect Ed, and we go upstairs to talk to Dr. D'Angelo. He is direct and sensitive. "This is not a viable pregnancy," he says. "This shell of an embryo looks as if it is about to crumple." He can perform a D and C or I can wait for it to pass naturally. As he speaks, he looks at me and cocks his head way over to one side in an acknowledgment of what is not being said. I was all right while the talk stayed clinical, but this gesture of kindness is too much for me.

It takes a moment or two for it to reach me, so that he is on to other medical talk when I begin to howl, to sob, to scream with sorrow, to turn my face away from my husband and my as-if doctor and loose all the rage and sadness and frustration of the past seven years. Ed races over to me from his chair and places his husbandly arms around me. It is my turn. His will come later. I will hold him and stroke his hair and tell him that I love him, that everything will be all right. But now he is here for me. The doctor winds up the session and tells us we can stay in his office as long as we need to. He closes the door behind him.

I stay there keening, wild with something primal, unable to gain any kind of composure. After a long time we leave. When I get home I find in my pocket the technician's report, the kind of report Dr. Gold always protected me from seeing:

*Transabdominal examination is performed and compared to recent prior studies. A small, somewhat irregular, poorly defined gestational sac is again noted. This is situated towards the region of the uterine body and lower uterine segment. Within this sac is an area of clumped echoes. No fetal cardiac activity is noted. If this did represent a fetal pole, its size would suggest an age of 6.5 weeks. By this time, cardiac activity should be witnessed. This may simply represent residual tissue and/or blood. In any case, a viable pregnancy is not demonstrated.*

In the first dream, a sweet-tempered young man from my office is a mentally impaired, potentially violent fellow who takes offense at an older man who is trying to calm him down. The younger man works up a tremendous spit, which he lets fly at close range in the other man's face. Suddenly Jack Nicholson appears as a coworker and has sharp words with the young man. Neither backs down. Then Jack opens a pair of scissors wide and solemnly tells the rest of us: "Call Security."

In another dream I am sitting around a table with a group of women while someone explains to us our choice. We have all lost a baby and are being given the option of having its body or its ashes returned to us. We all request ashes, except for one young woman, who wants the body. The blackish, decomposing torso of a child—without head or limbs—is handed to her. It looks bumpy, textured in some way, and she begins to squeeze and press on it, all quite lightheartedly. As she does, a fluid squirts out of the body, a fetid death juice that splashes into my face in such a tactile way that after jumping into a wakened state I wonder whether my cat may have urinated on me.

A third dream is not a nightmare but a vivid view of my own body from the point of view of an examining doctor. I clearly see my ovaries as large sacs containing many large, round eggs.

In the last dream, I give birth at four months. I have to be told that this is dangerous and unusual, and then explain it to Ed. Our daughter is in a room with many other newborns. I go in alone and know her right away—she looks a bit like me. But she is the size of a four- or five-year-old child, and her arms and legs hang out of the cradle they've put her in. Her head is bent straight back at the neck. I lift it, prepared for the worst, but she is quite alive and speaks to me, asking, "Mommy, what does 'pretty' mean?"

I refused Dr. D'Angelo's offer of a D and C. I wanted to miscarry on my own, the closest it seemed I would get to natural childbirth. Let it come, I thought, when it's ready.

Weeks passed, I somehow went about my work and my life, but still it clung. We waited it out, telling no one of our unspeakable predicament. When I explained to a nurse that I had

had two other miscarriages, both of them quick and one of them painless, she told me I'd been lucky. Yeah. Lucky.

Eventually I decided it would be macabre not to have a D and C performed. But where? Orphaned by my fertility center, having no gynecologist since I'd been a fertility patient for seven years, beginning to understand what it means to be someone with a long story, I sought out my old Manhattan gynecologist, Dr. Weintraub. I had come full circle.

Dr. Weintraub still had the picture of women's underwear in his office and still wore a large, dark toupee. I left his office after a preliminary checkup carrying an insurance statement that listed my condition as "fetal demise." The terminology stabbed me. Couldn't they come up with something more medical-sounding?

He still liked to perform his surgical procedures out of town, in the suburban facility where I had been Dr. Gold's patient. Its upper level still housed an abortion clinic. So, after trying to have a baby for seven years and making the excruciating decision to have the vestiges of a new life suctioned from my body, Ed and I had to pass a group of picketing antiabortionists on our way into the center. I thought about approaching them, just to explain how unimaginably complicated people's lives can become, but I wouldn't have known where to begin.

# Chapter 10

# Misconceptions

My bowling was lousy, but that was nothing new. I'd never been good at it, and had joined the bowling league only as a goof when my good buddy Mike suggested it: an excuse to get together with him for a few laughs every Monday night. But there was no laughter this night. Tears threatened to spill out every time I missed an easy spare. My tolerance for setbacks had been drained clean by Linda's third miscarriage, which had ended all hope of having a baby of our own.

As we took off our bowling shoes after the last game, Mike told me to forget about how I had played. "Who cares?" he said. "Bowling isn't real life, remember?" I shrugged. He couldn't guess what was going on in my "real life," because I had never told him that I'd been trying and failing to have a kid ever since I'd met him almost seven years ago.

A few months later I gave him the whole story, while we were having dinner at a Mexican restaurant. Maybe it was the margaritas that allowed me to blow my cover; he was the first person I'd mentioned the infertility to other than my immediate family and medical professionals. The pitch and volume of Mike's voice dropped as I relayed the series of low points to him, but he didn't have much to say. If someone had told me such news, I would have been rendered equally mute if I didn't have a similar history to reflect on. Mike was also probably stunned that I hadn't told him about the infertility years before. Maybe he thought that I harbored many secrets, that I didn't consider him such a close friend. That he didn't really know me at all.

I'd become a middle-aged man who by that time had expected to have one kid about six years old and another about three, but who had only a nine-year-old cat. I could hardly listen while male friends confessed going through a midlife crisis; my own had been either delayed or co-opted by my ongoing infertility. They fretted about gray hairs sprouting on the sides of their heads, or pulling muscles while running to first base. I had no gray and could still sprint down the line without injury, but I had a huge hollow space inside me that kept getting bigger.

It had been a precipitous fall since the beginning of the year, when Dr. Gold had talked to us about coming to California again for another procedure. The memory of our failed IVF eight months earlier was still fresh in our minds, but he wanted to try something different this time: gamete intra-fallopian transfer, known in the trade by the optimistic acronym of GIFT.

The timing for a new conception attempt had felt right to me, because it was going to take place a few weeks after I hit the big four-oh. I had this notion that forty would be the official beginning of a new era for me. I kicked off my new decade with a birthday party at a Manhattan pool hall that included among its guests four of my best boyhood friends, a couple of whom I hadn't seen in fifteen years. We feasted on memories of youthful shenanigans, laughed over pictures in high school yearbooks, and floated back to the days when everything seemed possible. Perhaps I wasn't that old after all, I thought. Perhaps this was the best time for me to become a father.

I added a positive note to our second trip west by tacking on a visit to my sister Chris's family in Arizona, where my parents would join us from New Mexico. Linda and I decided that we would drive to Los Angeles from there, taking a scenic route through the Grand Canyon, Utah, and Nevada.

Injecting Linda with drugs felt almost routine this time around, but it felt weird doing it at my sister's house. Hidden behind the closed door of my niece's bedroom, where we slept, I jabbed Linda under a lamp shaped like a duck while surrounded by Barbie dolls and stuffed animals. I imagined losing a syringe under the bed, and my sister finding it when she changed the sheets. Oh my God! she'd scream in horror. My daughter's a drug addict!

During the visit I was forced to address the topic of my infertility one day after playing tennis at a local health club with my father and brother-in-law, Hank. My father suggested we hop into the Jacuzzi, and I had to say no thanks. "Come on, Ed, this is great," said Hank as he slid into the steaming water. I shook my head. "Don't you like Jacuzzis?" asked my father. "I'm not supposed to go in them," I said. "Bad for sperm count."

My father averted his eyes. Hank squinted and nodded gravely as he looked over at me. "That has to be tough," he said. "How's everything going with that?"

Talking about my infertility in even this matter-of-fact way set something off in me, and I was grateful for the sunglasses hiding my eyes. Suddenly I felt inferior among these two men who had sired five children between them. I imagined them as tribesmen in a forest, spearing animals while I was relegated to gathering berries and kindling.

I considered telling them about our IVF debacle the previous year and the upcoming GIFT. I imagined my father's reaction if I told him that Linda and I had probably spent close to $10,000 trying to get a kid so far, when you factored in all the travel expenses. Jesus, he'd say; that's more than I paid for my car. I started talking about how great the weather was out in the Sun Belt.

The day before, Hank had asked me if I wanted to go on a bike ride. I had quietly declined that offer, too. Studies had shown that sitting on a bicycle seat for prolonged periods could kill sperm. I blocked my desire for a second cup of coffee in the morning or a second round of cocktails in the evening because I knew caffeine and alcohol could have some effect on the prostate gland, which played a key role in semen production. Every move I made was prescribed by my concern about my fertility.

While walking with Chris around the neighborhood one morning as a flock of quail sprinted across the street in front of us, I decided to tell her about the GIFT. I even mentioned the shots I'd been giving Linda under her roof. She seemed hungry for the news. Who knew what she had been thinking all those years? Soon after telling my parents about the infertility years before, I had written a letter to Chris about what Linda and I had been through. But I couldn't remember having brought up the subject with her again.

Chris echoed hope back to me as I filled her in, and I wondered why I had been so unwilling to talk to her about it. Then I knew. Now, whether the GIFT worked or not, I would later have to tell Chris how it went; I wouldn't be able to hide out with the news. While others in my situation might have been grateful to have people around who knew and would care if the procedure failed, I felt as if any sadness she sent my way would only deepen my own.

Soon I was eager to get out of Arizona, to escape the intense heat, avoid further questioning, and close the gap between us and Dr. Gold's magic touch. As we raced down the often empty highways on our way west, surrounded by mesas and desert, I once again allowed myself to feel that we were giving infertility the slip.

Linda responded well again to the Pergonal. I had no problems producing a sperm sample. Eggs and sperm took a ride together down Dr. Gold's miniature flume, through Linda's belly button, the same site where she had first been connected to her mother's life-support system. Dr. Gold also added our three thawed embryos left from the IVF into the mix.

After the surgery, all pretense of this being some sort of vacation ended. Linda had to recover. I propped her up with pillows in our hotel room as we foraged on room service meals and pay-per-view movies. I felt like we were hiding from the mob under the witness protection program. The only time we seemed to leave the room was to say prayers out by the pool, reciting tiny passages from a Mass card that Linda's sister had gotten for us on a trip to Rome. Neither of us had been to church in years, and I wasn't even Catholic, but by that point we were willing to embrace any faith or ritual that might help us. Not an hour would go by without my firing a missile of pleading skyward. I hoped my shotgun approach would catch the attention of whatever omnipotence might be up there. It didn't have to be God; at that point I would have sold my soul to Satan to get a child.

During the trip back home, we got a welcome dose of comic relief. I had to give Linda a shot of progesterone at regular intervals after the GIFT, and one came due during the time frame of our travel. There wasn't enough room in those casket-sized bathrooms on the plane for both of us to go in there and contort ourselves into position, so we'd have to take care of it at the Minneapolis airport where we'd be getting a connecting flight. We were trying to figure out how we might accomplish this when the solution presented itself: a self-enclosed, cubicle-size structure called a Ziosk. It was the state-of-the-art in accommodations for business travelers who had to work on the run, containing a phone, fax machine, hookups for computers, bed, and sink. Outside the Ziosk was a phone with a toll-free number listed for reserving it, and Linda called it. This was a new product, and the company that made it was as interested in promotion and getting information about us as in renting it out. Our flight to New York was leaving in twenty minutes.

"Listen to me," Linda said as the telemarketer droned on. "I've got to get in there right now, do you understand me?"

I figured there was no way we could cut through whatever bureaucratic crap was in our way, but Linda's authoritative stance managed to get us a booking immediately. We scanned our credit card through the slot in the door and in we went, armed not with briefcases and marketing reports but syringes and vials. As I prepared the shot, I wondered if any people who'd seen us thought we were going in there for a quickie. I had an urge to shake the walls of the place, to start groaning "Oh, yes!" as I pumped the drugs into Linda's right buttock, upper right quadrant.

When we got home, I kept my confidence in a tiny place in the back of my mind, occasionally allowing myself to remember that Dr. Gold said the procedure went especially well. When a pregnancy test showed up positive, I managed to feel that this pregnancy was more real than the previous one four years earlier, that the odds for success had improved through the three pregnancies. Linda told her family about it, but I had to take a step back from everyone's optimism. I didn't tell my sister or anyone in my family as the weeks of the pregnancy continued adding up, and wasn't sure how pregnant Linda had to be for me to speak up.

Since I'd never told my sister that Linda had gotten pregnant, I didn't have to tell her that she'd miscarried. I didn't tell her that she'd seen an obstetrician, so I didn't have to tell her how the obstetrician said everything looked fine the day before an ultrasound examination indicated otherwise.

I had stood there while a technician with little knowledge of fertility problems moved the ultrasound wand around inside Linda to find the heartbeat that was supposed to be there. She kept enlarging the image on the screen in search of the little blip we'd yet to see. I hoped that making it bigger would give the shape more chance of being alive, but it didn't. The image lost more and more detail, becoming an aerial view of a town, then a forest, then a vast desert, finally the surface of the moon.

* * *

I was continually on edge, as if the slightest stimulus would short-circuit me and make me collapse to the floor. Everything had sharp edges. Everyone had too much treble in their voices. Light coming toward me coalesced into beams that cut into me like Dr. Gold's lasers into Linda. Cars going by on the highway were tanks invading my neighborhood. I couldn't find pleasure in anything. I felt as though I was losing my past as well as my future. Birth certificates would be shredded, treasured family photos tossed into the fireplace.

When I went to malls and found myself surrounded by women and kids, kids, kids, I no longer saw myself as just an outsider, I felt dangerous to them. I cut a wide swath around babies in strollers and toddlers on foot, as if I was a carrier of doom to future generations.

Fears and superstitions dormant since childhood were resurrected. I had once had a theory that souls were passed on from parent to child, that this was the only ticket to immortality. The miscarriage had me fearing for my future in the universe. I sensed that I was closer to death myself, as if the Grim Reaper were working his way closer to me, to Linda, to my entire family.

I didn't know if my thoughts were normal for someone who'd been through what I'd been through, or just normal for *me*. I wondered if there were support groups for men going through this. Probably not; men hated to share their feelings. Men were supposed to attack their sorrow with a blowtorch, to bite a bullet until their teeth cracked to distract themselves from the emotional pain.

But I wasn't like other men. I wanted a kid more than they did. I wanted a kid more than Linda did, and always had. Did that mean I was suffering more than she was? Linda didn't yearn for tragedy, but she'd always had a better relationship with it than I did. She seemed to draw strength from its intensity. I couldn't accept it, tried to deny it was there or pretend it wasn't so bad. It just weighed me down and left me there.

The present was bleak, the future uncertain, so I traveled back in time. One afternoon I scaled the rickety ladder up to the sweltering attic in search of the suitcase holding my personal archives. I found it buried under a tent I hadn't slept in for fourteen years and a trombone I hadn't played in almost thirty. I hungrily pulled out the relics, coughing as the dust motes were sucked into my lungs, hearing droplets of sweat fall from my present onto my past. I spread out medals and trophies, report cards and term papers.

I gazed over and over at an old yearbook, not my high school one but an earlier one, from back when I was safe from any notions of sex or pregnancy or serious relationships or child-rearing. I looked long and hard at my thumb-sized fourteen-year-old face, waiting for it to talk to me, but it just sat there with its stupid smile sitting above a thin polyester tie and plaid sports jacket. I savored the superficial messages written by my classmates after my graduation. "Have a great summer. See you in high school." "Good luck to a great kid." I flipped to the picture of my girlfriend at the time. She'd drawn a heart around her face and made reference to some inside joke about a party we'd gone to. I'd never laid a finger on her except to make out. I didn't know I was supposed to.

Eventually real life hauled me back into the present. I began trying to look ahead to the option still left to Linda and me, which posed entirely different kinds of problems: adoption. It was like getting a new job I had absolutely no training for. But at least I was certain I wanted a child. Linda wasn't so sure. I had convinced myself that her ambivalence would fade as we got closer to the prize, but we hadn't talked about it much.

Private adoption was a complicated and expensive process that involved hiring a lawyer, submitting documents to the state that proved you weren't a child abuser, being evaluated by a social worker, and finding a birth mother who wanted to give up her child. Most disturbing of all was how birth mothers were typically found: by running classified ads in newspapers.

At an adoption conference, we discovered that all sorts of businesses had sprung up to accommodate the growing pool of couples looking to adopt. There were counselors who advised parents before and after they adopted, companies specializing in international adoption. Even adoption termination insurance, which compensated couples for the expenses of an adoption that fell through.

We got the name of an attorney who specialized in private adoption. "Let me tell you this," he said from across what seemed like a football field–sized desk in his spacious office as we kept sinking in his cushy leather chairs. "You two are going to adopt a baby. Follow the steps I give you, and you'll be parents before very long." I felt giddy with hope as the lawyer continued talking, especially since I'd already heard that he had a reputation for plugging up all the loopholes, cutting red tape with a wave of his hand, and sniffing out fraudulent birth mothers like a bloodhound.

Unfortunately, babies made their way to childless couples like us on a road paved with gold. Before the attorney made one move in our cause, we had to give him a retainer of $700. Then we had to fork out another $600 for a home study: a visit to our house by a social worker who would judge our worthiness as parents and the quality of our home as an environment for a child.

The retainer to the attorney gave us the privilege of doing tons of work ourselves. He would have no involvement with us again until we found a child to adopt—a process that could take months, even years. Apparently there were legal restrictions against attorneys helping couples find a child to adopt.

After filling out various forms, we needed to prove that our faces shouldn't be on Wanted posters at the post office. This involved going to a local police station to get fingerprinted, so they could make sure we didn't have a criminal record. I walked in there feeling twinges of guilt, as if they'd slam the cuffs on me for plotting to steal a baby. But the officer who inked our fingers was nice. He joked about how he was going to grill us under a hot light before he let us go.

In preparation for the home study, we cleaned our house as it had never been cleaned before. Then we spent time prepping each other so we'd be ready to talk at length about our idyllic childhoods, warm marriage, emotional stability, unshakable job security, and ability to provide the most enriching childhood available in the 1990s.

When the social worker arrived, my expectations of being put on the defensive turned out to be way off the mark. Her matter-of-fact tone made it easy to answer questions about our life together ("We're best friends," I said) and how infertility affected our marriage ("It's made our bond even stronger," Linda said). Jokes were tossed back and forth, laughter echoed off the walls. She nodded perfunctorily when we showed her the room designed for the baby, jotting down notes on her legal pad. Her visit seemed like a mere formality.

Although the home study report gave us the thumbs-up, we held off trying to find a birth mother. Linda wasn't ready to make a move. I'll never forget what happened one night when, sitting at the kitchen table, she asked, "Are you sure you want to go through with this? It's a completely different thing than having your own child."

"There's no other way," I said as I wiped off the butcher-block top on the island. "I don't like the process either. But how else can we get a child?"

Linda closed her eyes and shook her head.

"I'm not just talking about *how* it's done," she went on, trying hard to maintain a level tone. "I simply don't know if I can go through with it. I'm afraid about how I might feel about the child."

I'd tried to push my recognition of Linda's thoughts about adoption out of my mind, but of course I hadn't; I had only stored them somewhere. When she brought up her concerns, a new Pandora's box of fears in me was opened. Fears about what all those years of struggle had done, fears about the future. How could I still believe that a baby would miraculously dissolve the buildup of negative feelings from all those years? Linda was finally balking at taking the next step, but I had no plan or means for dealing with it because I'd never allowed it as a possibility.

My hands became glued to the butcher block. I couldn't sit down next to Linda, couldn't move any closer to her, couldn't even look at her. We were beyond the point where I could tell her that I was sure she'd love being a mother, or that she was just stressed out from the infertility. This was bigger than all of those things, and it had created a vast space between us in that room.

Why had I allowed myself to hide from this lack of unity between us? Maybe because my passive aggressiveness had worked too often in the past. How many times over the years had I gotten my way not by fighting for it, but by remaining mute? Linda had wanted to stay in New York after we first met, but she moved to the suburbs to be with me. She'd wanted to delay getting married, but we didn't. She'd wanted a small wedding, but didn't get one. She hadn't been sure she wanted kids, but we'd spent the better part of a decade struggling against all odds to have one. I'd surrounded myself with a shield of silence, letting Linda's objections bounce off until she gave up. It was the behavior of a child who closed his eyes to make an unpleasant scene around him disappear.

I knew that if this had been a debate, Linda would have won. On her side were years of medical invasions, despair, failure, and money down the drain. I could promise only the possibility of a new kind of fulfillment in the future. But my claims carried no weight. Was I any different from a cult leader telling someone to commit suicide because heaven was so wonderful?

Or was Linda the one being unreasonable after all? I wanted to be a father, but now I felt I had to prove it was important to me. Why should I have had to? Hell, I was the norm in wanting kids and Linda was the rebel.

I was paralyzed. Whatever was going through my head seemed impossible to translate into words. I felt that anything I said would be incomprehensible, even to me.

"I don't know what I'm supposed to say," I said after a long silence. I darted a glance at Linda, relieved that I didn't make eye contact.

"I've tried to imagine not being a father. You know what I've come up with? Becoming a movie star. Or a rock star. It's ridiculous, I know. It's not going to happen. But it's like, if I don't have a child, I have to make sure that I'm immortal in some way."

"You make it sound like your whole life so far has been meaningless," Linda said. "And you're still only talking about *you.* What about *us*? Ed, don't you see that what we've gone through has taken something away from us that we can't get back?"

I couldn't bear to ask what that "something" was. I still insisted on sidestepping bad news, even though I was waist-deep in it. Our future child seemed to be in the room with us at that moment. I could hear someone else breathing, shuffling on the carpet. I was trapped in the middle, loyal to both parties, but one party was the love of my life, standing in front of me right now, and the other wasn't even born yet.

Even now, when my marriage and my last stab at fatherhood were under fire, I didn't know what to say. I held back the tears. I stared out the window, where there was only darkness. Finally, Linda agreed that she wouldn't rule out adoption, as long as we went to see a counselor to discuss it first. Once again, I had brought her to my side by silence. I knew it was unfair, that the issue hadn't been resolved in the slightest. But I simply had no other resources to draw on.

* * *

A few days later, after I dropped Linda off to catch her morning train, some of the things she'd said to me that night began to resurface. Perhaps because I couldn't bear to hear them come from her, they were lip-synched by someone else: Dr. Flexner. His image began bombarding me with questions, like a ventriloquist's dummy turned devil's advocate. And he insisted on delving deeper than I had allowed Linda to.

"Are you sure you really want kids?" he asked.

"Yes, of course," I said.

"Couldn't it be another example of your relentless, often misguided pursuit of goals?"

"What goals?"

"How about the time you swam the entire length of your town pool underwater, even though you developed a splitting headache and almost passed out with forty feet left to go?"

"I was twelve years old!"

"Or the time you kept holding yourself up on that chinning bar, until the pain was so great you actually ejaculated?"

"I was only fourteen."

"Or how about that woman you proposed to before you met Linda? You would've married her. You would have spent your life with her, whether it was good for you or not."

"I thought she was the one."

"You thought? You didn't think at all, that's the point. You *decided* that's what you were going to do, therefore absolving yourself from having to think about it."

"That's absurd. Besides, we didn't get married."

"Only because *she* said she wasn't sure. She wanted to think it over, and only because of that you gave yourself *permission* to think about the relationship. Only then did you realize that you'd been fooling yourself about that relationship, that she was not right for you and never had been."

"Are you saying I'm fooling myself about wanting to be a father?"

"A long time ago you decided that you wanted a kid, that you'd make a great father. No amount of pain or hardship seems able to stop you. You're willing to give up every cent and everything else good in your life to get that child. Does that make sense to you?"

On the way back to my house I became aware that my foot was pushing the accelerator almost to the floor, my tires screeching as I barely stayed on the winding road. Was my whole life a big lie? Had I rationalized a series of wrong decisions about my career, how I wanted to live my life, even about Linda?

I began looking for hints that Linda and I really weren't right for each other. Was it significant that I loved to do crossword puzzles but she didn't? That I preferred the wilderness while she preferred the city? That I hated almost every pair of shoes she'd ever bought? Even now I was resorting to jokes to bail myself out. A classic male response: prevent yourself from having to reflect too much by making light of it. Enlightenment upstaged by entertainment.

My ability to judge anything large or small seemed under question. If I could just shake the stress out of me and think with a clear head. I would have liked to share some of these thoughts with Linda, but I couldn't make sense of them myself and was too afraid that her response to them would just widen the rift.

I had to figure out a way to make this all work out. I revived the old logic: having a kid was part of the big picture, essential for a full life, and Linda had to be part of that life. I couldn't give up the hope that she ultimately wanted this, too. I saw myself at the blackboard in school, writing down a hundred times what I desperately needed to be true: "Linda really wants this as much as I do. Linda really wants this as much as I do."

I drove past our street. I thought maybe I'd keep driving, head north until I ran out of gas. But I went home after about ten miles, too tired to focus on the road. I wanted to shift into reverse in my life. I wanted to go back to before Linda and I even started trying to conceive. I wanted to go back to the day we first passed each other at work, neither of us knowing the other's name but both turning our heads to give the other a second look as we continued down the corridor. Then I wanted to go back further, to get back to the root of all this, of myself, back to my childhood to see why I'd become this obsessive person. I couldn't tell whether I'd been turned neurotic by the pressures of infertility, or whether the neurosis had always been in me, had always been ruling my life but in less dramatic fashion.

A few weeks later Linda and I met with a therapist she had found out about in a newsletter put out by *Resolve* that dealt with infertility and adoption. Within a few minutes of our first session, adoption had become almost a side issue. All it took was a few questions about my family, and the therapist was digging away at my past. He was skeptical of my claims of a blissful childhood. He thought I must be hiding from something, or protecting myself against some painful truth. First Dr. Flexner, then

Dr. Holman, now this guy. The pattern was becoming clearer: I was a man who worked very hard at not really knowing himself. I came up with explanations for myself that held up logically but that used only some elements of my life story.

We stopped going to the therapist after a few sessions—not because he wasn't good, but because maybe he was too good. I think we were both afraid that we might end up hearing an "in-" word much more ominous than infertility: "incompatibility."

In the fall of 1994, we finally began getting down to the "business" part of finding a baby. Linda felt uncomfortable with this process, so it was all up to me. I tried to shift my perspective to that of the marketing professional I was, pretending I was doing the job for a client and not myself. I pored over the guidelines laid out in a book about adoption that our lawyer himself had written. I got a new phone line with a toll-free number that could be included in our adoption ads. Then I went to the library and found a directory of newspapers, writing down dozens of them from all over the country.

The chapter on writing ads had said it was important to start it with an "A" word, since ads were often listed alphabetically. I toyed with various combinations, testing my powers of alliteration. I finally settled on "Abundant affection awaits . . ." as an opener, following with a concise combination of parental virtues that we could offer a child. Then I earmarked ten newspapers from my master list, picking them more or less at random.

I called newspapers I'd never read in places I'd never been. Some people who answered my calls were supportive, wishing me good luck and even telling me which days were best for running ads in their papers (the ones with coupons had especially high readership). Others told me with disdain that their paper didn't allow such ads, making it clear that they thought "buying babies" was despicable. I wanted to tell them that I didn't want to get a baby this way, that it was the only way someone like me could do it, but they hung up on me before I could say anything else.

I faxed the ad and my credit card information to daily papers in Milwaukee and St. Louis. To *Pennysavers* in South Bend, Indiana, and Erie, Pennsylvania. To papers with a huge circulation where ad space cost plenty and ones with a small circulation where ad space cost peanuts. I kept a careful tally of our expenses in a three-ring binder in which I glued states cut out from a *Rand McNally Road Atlas* and circled the towns being targeted. I was an air force general mapping out bombing missions.

A new confidence filled me. I expected lots of replies. After all, I was a direct response copywriter. I'd written ads that had sold everything from stroke-prevention drugs, to romance novels, to hats with birds crocheted on them. Why not this?

I imagined thousands of papers with our ad tossed onto front porches by boys on bicycles, thousands more being snapped up outside kiosks on city streets and in train stations. Who would call us? I wondered. A teenage girl who got pregnant in the back of the limo with her prom date? A divorced mother of five on welfare? A fast-track single executive?

Then I was deflated when I saw our ads on the torn-out pages sent to us by the newspapers. Our postage stamp of a plea seemed inconsequential surrounded by so much newsprint, so many distractions. Our search for a child was buried among offers of cars for sale, announcements of upcoming tag sales, opportunities to meet single white males in their forties who enjoyed romantic dinners and waterskiing. Even worse, our ad was seldom the only one seeking a baby.

Soon Linda was back in the loop, because I never answered our toll-free phone; we'd read that most birth mothers prefer talking to women. I wondered at first if Linda's ambivalence would affect her phone manner. "So you had a baby," I imagined her saying to a caller in a monotone voice. "I guess we'll take it. Whatever." But Linda played her role perfectly. She was warm, sincere, and patient with every caller—even with the ones who obviously just wanted to talk and talk, at our expense.

There were calls from women who seemed intent on giving us their baby but never called back. From a woman who wanted to be a surrogate for *my* child ("Could you just mail out the sperm to me?" she actually said). Even a man called once, telling us about a "friend" who was in trouble.

After round three and having spent over $3,000 for our bite-sized pleas, we heard from Nellie: a pregnant, sixteen-year-old junior in high school who'd seen our ad in an Omaha daily. She told Linda that another couple had promised to adopt her baby but then had backed out. She was eight and a half months along and needed to find an adoptive couple fast.

I was bubbling with nervous excitement. There were more calls from Nellie in the days that followed, and I hungrily consumed every fact about her and the baby that Linda told me. She was an adoptive couple's dream birth mother; we'd get the baby fast, without the emotional and financial entanglements of a lengthy, dubious wait.

How ironic that Linda was the one making it all happen now. She handled the calls with Nellie so well that I was almost able to believe that her mixed feelings about adoption had faded. Meanwhile, I convinced myself that our ad had struck something deep in this teenager, that she had felt we were reaching out personally to her and just her. Luck had to be finally turning our way after all we'd been through. How could Linda not jump on board in the face of such a fortuitous turn of events? Someday she'd say to me, "I can't believe I had my doubts about adopting." I kept telling myself this louder and louder in my head, working hard to drown out the other voices that were fighting for airtime.

# Chapter 11

# Grounds for Marriage

The few times over the years when I tried to discuss my hesitation about the fertility treatment, or just blow off steam, a look of such despair spread over Ed's face that I couldn't bring myself to do it. It was easier to sign up for the next surgery. Between Ed and Dr. Gold, I could have kept going forever.

But we'd decided that the medical battle was over. We'd lost. Not too many years earlier, the battle would barely have been fought at all. Ed and I would have had a few visits with my gynecologist, maybe a primitive pill to coax my ovaries into higher performance, or surgery to remove my endometrial cyst, then watched the baffled doctor shake his head and shrug his shoulders as he admitted that he really couldn't say what was wrong; had we considered adoption? We'd have faced it fast, before our differences and our desires had had time to harden into obsessions, into camps.

Modern medicine is sophisticated enough to offer micromanipulation of sperm, pre-implantation genetic testing, and donor eggs—it's already offering things not dreamed of even in the early nineties, when Ed and I went high-tech—but modern men and women are no more sophisticated than our historical counterparts. We can't all sort through the medical possibilities and come up with a workable ethic for ourselves. Half of infertile couples will have a baby with a doctor's help. Some will adopt. Others will live out their lives without children. Still others may divorce.

My husband crossed smoothly over into the idea of adoption, as though it were just the next step with Dr. Gold. I'd become somewhat obsessed with the battle along the way, too, but I kept certain distinctions clear in my mind. Trying to outsmart our bodies' refusal to procreate with a doctor's help was one thing. Accepting into our home a child who'd come from donor sperm or a birth mother called on an entirely different set of muscles.

Deep down, I guess I never thought it would really come to that. Adoption. The word connoted illicit love, abandonment, poverty. When I was a kid, wondering what lay in store and how I'd deal with various circumstances, I would think, "Yeah, I guess I'll have children if I marry. But if I can't get pregnant, I wouldn't adopt." In the same way, I'd thought if I'd turned out to be, say, lesbian, I'd deal with it; I wouldn't be too happy about it, but I'd deal with it.

Well, I grew up straight and I got married, but I wasn't able to make a baby. This is where I was supposed to stop. I wasn't proud of the fact that I couldn't embrace adoption, and I was certainly happy for people who did, but it was a leap of faith I wasn't sure I was up to. It was no easier broaching the subject of my hesitation about adoption with Ed than it had been my hesitation about the fertility treatments. Were we done mourning the biological child we probably wouldn't have? Who knows? How many tears are enough? I'd been through a miscarriage three times, my body fighting against what it was designed to do. When I thought that three times a tiny mass existed that was a combination of Ed and me, that it had had the blueprint for specific, real features, for a certain personality, my throat would catch and my breath would stop. "Hell," I'd have to convince myself at those times, drawing on my waning cynicism, "they just grow up and break your heart."

Somewhere along the line, though, there had been a consensus: we would do whatever it took to have a baby. Medically. Financially. Emotionally. How is it that I had tacitly agreed to that? And why couldn't I speak up to say it was time to stop?

It went deeper than that. How do a man and woman come together as a committed couple? They don't just fall for each other. They *sense* certain things about the other person, things they're not consciously aware of, things that won't come into play for years. One couple we're close with were both hardworking professionals when we met them. But when the first of three children arrived twelve years ago, she quit work and has been home with them ever since; he's gotten higher- and higher-paying jobs all that time. And I know a corporate lawyer whose husband stays home with the kids. Somehow these couples knew they would provide that to each other when the time came.

So how come Ed picked me? A woman whom he knew felt ambivalent about having children at all, let alone setting records to make it happen. What wires were getting crossed when he remained convinced he wanted suburbia and parenthood while falling in love with me and wanting to marry me? And me, too. If I pictured myself independent and urban for the rest of my life, how'd I wind up with someone whose self-image revolved around fatherhood? And how on earth had I made my way through all the drama and turmoil of fertility treatment as though I'd had no choice but to follow it through to the end?

I began to think that couples who were married and happy were just married and untested. Maybe they just hadn't come across real trouble yet. Ed and I'd been happy because we both wanted the same thing for so long: each other. And I always thought we were very much alike. It was easy to compromise because neither had to budge that far to get to the compromise point. But Ed's mandate for fatherhood changed all that. I wanted him at least to acknowledge that it had become an obsession, that not everybody would be willing to risk everything for it.

I told my friend Kathleen one day that Ed and I were getting ready to proceed with adoption plans even though I had mixed feelings. The engine was already running; I didn't feel it was in my power to stop it. We should at least, my friend said with alarm, see a counselor together before taking such a big step. Her simple, rational reaction gave me the strength I needed to conjure up a confrontation with Ed. The ridiculous truth was that in our fifteen years together, we'd rarely had one. But we did that night. I'll never forget it.

When I get home from work, I bring up the topic. As usual, Ed's face takes on an expression so pained that my immediate instinct is to back off. But this time I persist. I need him, just this once, to hear me. If we lose honesty and open communication as a basis for our marriage, what will we have left? Am

I going too far in helping him adopt, farther than I have any right to go, so far as to be irresponsible?

"When?" I ask Ed. "When are we going to be able to talk about this? Am I allowed to say that I don't think I want to adopt? Will you at least *acknowledge* what I'm thinking?"

He's not looking at me. He's busying himself with the dinner preparations. My rational, measured reactions, piling up year after year, now flood out as anger. I need to hurt him.

"What the hell do we think we're doing, for God's sake? We're about to sink thousands of dollars into a weird process that ends when we take home another woman's child? And we can't even *talk* about the fact that I don't feel right about it?"

"We can talk, we can talk," he replies, struggling with a colander. "Go ahead and talk." Still he won't look at me.

"Ed, I don't think I can go through with it." I have needed so badly to say those words out loud. Suddenly I am immense, while Ed shrinks before my eyes. I continue. "It's one thing to find out what's wrong with us physically that's stopping me from getting pregnant. But to track down a stranger through want ads, to put our future in the hands of a lawyer . . . Why isn't it handled through a social worker?"

"I don't like the process either, but that's how it has to be done."

"I don't like the process, or the whole idea. We can't have a baby. Why can't we just move on with our lives?"

Ed is bringing our plates over to the table, but I know I won't be able to take a bite.

"This is enough for you? Just the way things are now?" he asks me. He just can't accept that I'm not feeling what he is.

"Yes, goddammit! I don't feel any void! This is my life! I like my life!"

My heart is racing. I am raising my voice and not sure where it is all leading. I'm on the verge of something that has to be said, though I don't know what it is yet.

"Ed, what if we do this thing, and then find I can't ever forget that the kid isn't ours? What if I can't live like that?" Then it comes out before I have a chance to think it first: "Do you think you can raise a child alone?"

The words hang in the kitchen between us. My gauntlet. My last straw.

After a moment Ed says dryly, as close to bitter as I have ever seen him: "I'll do what I have to do." Now he is looking me straight in the eye.

I hadn't even allowed myself to think it before that moment: my husband needs a child more than he needs me. I am not the love of his life, only the means through which he will come by it. Maybe I had never issued an ultimatum because I feared I might not win.

Before the infertility, we would have joked our way out of this; we would have gone through instinctual steps that made sure we'd come out on the same side. But we weren't on the same side anymore.

My throat is dry and constricted. I want more than anything to put my arms around my shy, nervous husband, the one I always go to for help, this suffering man whose heart I will break, whose heart I will lose, if I tell him I have reached my limit. Instead, I walk out of the room. I feel dizzy, stricken. The price of honesty.

In an instant I feel his arms around me, feel his warm tears on my neck. This is why I hadn't brought up my true feelings about the fertility treatments year after year. This is what I knew would happen.

I tuck Ed's head into my shoulder and stroke the back of his neck. I do love this man. It had never occurred to me that we might actually part over this. What kind of cute, irrelevant ride had I been on as my marriage, the only thing I really had, began to go slack from inattention, to stay fixed when it needed to bend? Fantasizing about having an affair with my doctor? Turning something sad and stressful into an opportunity to be a star? Why hadn't I spoken up more forcefully before now? What was wrong with me, with us, that we had allowed ourselves to get to this state unchecked? What did we *need*?

We had left an escape hatch open upon entering the state of matrimony: if I didn't come around to wanting children, Ed would presumably find someone who did. Was that grounds for marriage, no matter how much in love we were? What right did we have to do that to each other?

I stood in the hallway and comforted my husband. Where was *my* comfort going to come from?

I didn't know. And I didn't know whether I wanted to be an adoptive mother. All I knew was that the man I loved and had been married to for twelve years was weeping on my shoulder because I was denying him his last chance to be a father.

I had had my say. There was nothing left but to search for a baby to adopt. I would do this for my husband.

I won one battle, though: that of time. We'd decided to move out of my cousin's home after six years there, and I insisted that it made more sense to get settled someplace new before getting involved in an adoption. I was talking more to my friends about the predicament. Once the heavy weight of secrecy was lifted, it was much easier to see the dividing line between planning for the future and just plain neurosis.

Ed fretted: we were getting older; if we moved back to the city, it might be less appealing to a potential birth mother; we could see a counselor about it, but couldn't make a health insurance claim in case an adoption investigation fingered us as psychos. "Enough!" I finally shouted. "Christ! You've turned into a nutcase, Ed. Let's just take one thing at a time. We're moving first."

And so we did. We ruled out moving back to the city: too difficult and expensive with a child in the picture. By chance, by design, by joke, we wound up buying a house five minutes from Dr. Gold's old office. Ed began the arduous process of finding a birth mother. And I found myself getting excited by the possibility.

My notion of family had undergone a change that helped me take the step toward adoption. A few months after we moved into our new house, I made a trip to Florida to be with my mother on her seventieth birthday. Both of my sisters were there, too—no one's husband or kids, just the original five of us. We took Mom out for dinner, then stood talking in my parents' dining room after taking some Polaroids. One of my sisters put her arm around my mother, and I, on the other side, did the same. My other sister drifted over, and finally we beckoned my father to join the impromptu circle. And there we stood, interlocked, silent, beaming at one another, exuding a sense of well-being I couldn't remember ever feeling among that group in all my thirty-nine years. It was as if we'd been given one moment to reconcile and then would never see each other again. I wouldn't have been surprised to look down and find that we had levitated off the floor.

To think that after all the misunderstanding and harshness, the dislocation and disaffection, something new and good could come out of that circle was a revelation to my jaded sense of family. I had a fleeting thought that it was too bad I wasn't going to be able to contribute to the continuation of the line. After a long moment the circle was broken, but the feeling of a healed family, of family as something I would want to be part of, would stay with me.

When the calls from birth mothers started to come in, I was prepared. These were people who needed someone to talk to about a problem. I'd always been good in that role. My nervousness wore off after the first couple of talks, and then I enjoyed them. All I had to do was listen sympathetically and see where the conversations took us. Many of the women (and the occasional man) were simply grateful to have someone's attention and sympathy for an hour. Some of them called in the middle of the night. None of them called a second time.

Until Nellie. My first conversation with her, on a Saturday afternoon in March 1995, had been neither the longest nor the best of the dozen or so I'd had by then. But she called again the next day and said she wanted us to be the parents of her baby. Ed and I allowed ourselves a new and lovely happiness. The lawyers and other professionals had taken over behind the scenes, but onstage Nellie and I talked to each other just about every day in the two weeks that remained of her pregnancy.

She was much more mature than I'd been at sixteen, and I liked her honesty and strength. She was still driving forty-five minutes each way to a grocery-store job after school and on weekends. It didn't sound as though anyone at home was helping her through this, but her mother and stepfather, she said enthusiastically, were supportive. They were divorced and lived apart. Nellie's mother, at thirty-two, was seven years younger than I was, and only weeks earlier had had a baby with her estranged husband. The child we were going to adopt would have an uncle in the same grade at school.

When Nellie started having contractions, she called to let us know. She said she was uncomfortable, but sounded fearless. This was a girl who planned on finishing high school and going on to college. She had made a mistake somewhere along the way, on a heady June night under the bright Nebraska stars, judging by her due date, and meant to do right by this child.

Happily out of the closet, Ed and I shared the news with friends and family. This was *easy*. This was going to be the good part. In forty-eight hours, we put together the baby's room, stocked it with Pampers, then packed a suitcase for ourselves, filled another with baby clothes, and hauled out my sister's old infant car seat. When we got the word that Nellie had delivered a boy—nine pounds, six ounces—we were ecstatic.

"And now," my sister Barbara said during one of a score of phone calls I had with my sisters, my mother, my friends, my coworkers, that day, "now it's time to go pick up your son."

# Chapter 12

## Parental Discretion

She was bigger than I had expected, and not because she had just had a baby. I had imagined her small, weak, as if only frail girls would get pregnant while still in high school. Instead, she was almost six feet tall and brawny, her shorts stretched to the limit by the distended abdomen that had recently housed a nine-and-a-half-pound boy.

Linda and I were meeting Nellie in a small Nebraska town, not really a town at all but a place trapped between country and city, farm and factory. Buildings that looked like large packing crates lined the main drag between fast-food outlets and car dealerships. A few blocks to the left and right, and then there was nothing but dirt and scraggly bushes as far as we could see. Even though there wasn't a cloud in the sky when we arrived, it seemed as if the whole town were in shadow. As if the sun were turning itself into a black hole to avoid shedding light down onto this desolate, flat place where the wind filled the air with dust and the streets leading out of town headed nowhere.

We had taken a flight the day before to Denver, then driven two hundred miles north, because there was only a tiny airport within fifty miles of the town and only small planes landed there. No kid of mine was going into some single-engine Sky King job that got swallowed up by the tiniest cloud and pushed around by every little breeze. My wife's best friend had been killed in a plane like that, and I wanted to show God that we had learned our lesson well.

We checked into a small motel and asked the proprietor for a crib. She gave us one without asking why there was no baby with us. Arrive without a child, leave *with* a child? Maybe she'd think we were kidnappers.

Nellie didn't arrive at our meeting alone; her mother's ex-husband was with her. She lived with him instead of her mother, for reasons we didn't want to know. I thought maybe he was the baby's father, a case of incest-in-law, then put it out of my mind. Or put it somewhere in my mind where I couldn't see it for now. I had become good at that.

The stepfather was a cowboy, but no Gene Autry. Under his ten-gallon hat were a face and nose so red a bull would've charged at him. Perhaps he'd had too much sun and too much Wild Turkey. When I saw the volleyball he had under his cowboy shirt I changed my guess of whiskey to beer. He was so bowlegged you could have tossed a beach ball through his legs without touching denim. "We'll draw for it," I imagined him saying as he handed me a loaded Colt .45 and gestured for me to come outside.

Linda and I had met the baby less than an hour earlier. "Nellie's making the right decision," one of the nurses at the hospital told us. "He's the most well-behaved baby here," another one said. A model baby. Perhaps only a model of a baby, I thought. Just a symbol, a picture of a kid on Gerber products.

Then I saw him. He did look perfect. Strong, robust. I didn't want to touch him right away; I wanted to stare at him, sharpen my focus, freeze-frame him so he couldn't move out of my view ever again. I was incredulous rather than happy. No, it wasn't that. I'd been conditioned to fear elation, because over the past eight years it had always been followed by disappointment, and I didn't want to set up the same sequence. Only after looking at Linda's smiling face could I admit to myself that yes, it was okay to be a little happy now.

They let us sit alone in a room with him. A chance to bond. We looked at him, looked at each other, then at him again. We passed him back and forth as if practicing handoffs for a football game, mindful to support the head because the neck was too weak. "This is the real thing, right?" I asked Linda. She nodded vigorously and giggled, seeming twenty years younger. I felt that she and I were completely unified in the moment, our differences about adoption melting away.

A nurse came back. "Do you want to feed him?" she asked. Linda brought the bottle up to his mouth. He started spitting up, choking, and I felt helpless, as if the baby were in serious trouble. Then a nurse suctioned the spit-up from the baby's mouth with a bulb syringe. He was fine, not crying, didn't know anything had gone wrong. I settled down again, starting a relaxation exercise. *Breathe slowly. Relax toes. Relax feet.*

Having seen the baby began to seem unreal when we met Nellie's lawyer a half hour later. After five minutes of banter with him that was translated into gibberish the instant it entered my ears, he ushered Linda and me and Nellie into a conference room. We were to talk in there. No ground rules. Talk about what? What kind of music do you like, Nellie? Is it always this windy in Nebraska? Nellie kept folding and unfolding her hands across the table from us. I couldn't get over how big she was—the image I had of her in my head refused to give sway.

"Do you have any questions?" Nellie asked. I had none, but it didn't matter because she wouldn't look at me, didn't care one whit when Linda told her that we would be dividing the parenting duties fifty-fifty. Why should she? Some guy she'd never see again was the father of her child, and if I became the next father she would never see me again either.

"I'm a little confused," she suddenly said. "I have a friend who kept her baby and she wants me to keep mine." Every word she uttered dropped the temperature of the room another degree. Meanwhile, her stepfather or lover or rapist or whoever he was didn't give a shit either way; he was out in the hallway, probably yukking it up with the lawyer over the previous night's Jay Leno monologue.

"I don't know," Nellie said, her voice quavering. I couldn't think of anything to say. Our whole future was in her hands. But of course *her* future was in her hands, too. If I'd been plugged into my biofeedback device then, its pitch would've soared out of hearing range in seconds. I smiled faintly at Nellie, but she wasn't looking; I could have been making monkey faces, and it would still have been, Yes, thank you, you're very nice, sorry about all this.

We left the conference room. After we told the lawyer that Nellie wanted to think things over, his casual demeanor went rigid. "I didn't realize there would be any delay," he told us. Meanwhile a baby remained in a hospital ward, thinking his family was a group of paid medical professionals.

We called the lawyer the next morning. "She hasn't decided yet," he said. We told each other this was a good sign. We made plans to call the lawyer that evening and decided that we couldn't stand to remain in this town while waiting for the wind to blow the tumbleweeds one way and our fate the other. We hopped into our rented minivan and headed north, eager to get into another state. I thought maybe we could make it to the site of Custer's Last Stand in Montana, but it was too far, a two-day trip. What the hell, I thought; it was probably a tourist trap with ice cream places called Custard's Last Stand and restaurants serving Little Bighorn Burgers.

En route to the Black Hills of South Dakota we saw a highlighted area on our map, a museum on a site where they'd dug up dinosaur bones and you could walk around and look at them. It was hard for us to make the shift to tourist as we had in California during the IVF trip; I felt like an impostor as I gazed down at the giant ribs and pelvises. Lots of kids were there, their tiny hands safely enveloped within the hands of their parents. I prevented myself from picturing my hand holding anything so precious; such images had a tendency to turn into ghosts. I used to imagine a little girl skipping across my backyard, a girl who looked a lot like me. By the third miscarriage I had my imagination well trained and saw no one in my yard, nor anyone holding my hand, just my hand swaying next to me, occasionally tensing into a fist so tight that blood would ooze out from under my thumbnail.

We left the museum before the tour was over and headed for the hills again, the Black Hills, in hopes of escape, revelation. Anything. But we got there too late; the sun was setting fast, and there was barely time to see anything. Just silhouettes of deer or antelope against the orange sky.

We got back to the motel about seven-thirty. We walked in silently, in a state of mourning already, inoculating ourselves against the sorrow that might come out of that phone receiver. I wished that Linda would say something funny, or that I would, or that we could even recognize what was funny anymore. "I'll make the call," I said, then wished I hadn't. The calls I'd made that were infertility- or adoption-related totaled well into the triple figures by then. Doctors, laboratories, therapists, lawyers, newspapers, airlines, motels, car rentals. This was my job, and it was a bad one.

I called the number. The lawyer answered. "How did your day go?" he asked. A bad sign; no intro was ever required for good news. "She's going to keep him," he told me. I stared at the wall without blinking, perhaps incapable of ever blinking again. It was like hearing someone had died, although I knew the child was alive and well. But *our* child had died. "When did she call you?" I asked. "Late this afternoon. I think she's making the wrong choice. But as her attorney I can't tell her that." I was too numb to appreciate the irony that Linda and I were paying for this attorney's services, that he'd pick up a couple of grand from us for the privilege of telling us the last thing we wanted to hear.

I wanted to hate Nellie, but I couldn't. It was her baby—of course she should keep him. She was just a kid; she hadn't seen this coming. I held the phone to my ear for a long time after the lawyer hung up, waiting for him to come back on the line and tell me it was a mistake.

Finally I turned to Linda. She still held vague hope in her eyes, but too much time went by before I spoke, and she surmised the worst. I started thinking about all the emotional energy pumped into this trip and wondered if I would ever be able to get excited about anything again. The two of us were suddenly very alone in that room, unable to touch each other, even to look at each other.

I lay on the bed. The crib stared at me like a jail cell someone had broken out of, someone who would never be recaptured. The remote sat in my limp hand as I watched some bad movie on TV. No channel-surfing today like at home; I didn't have the energy to push a single button.

We left early the next morning. Boring landscape accompanied us for a hundred miles, our silence in the car accentuating the starkness. The scenery kept repeating, like in those cartoons where Wile E. Coyote pursues the Road Runner. An occasional grain silo or convenience store, otherwise flat dirt fanning out in every direction. Ground zero after the blast.

Somewhere near Council Bluffs, I felt the seat shaking. I stopped the car to hold Linda as she wept. I hugged her tightly, as if trying to squeeze out the sadness. Her pattern of sorrow was all too familiar to me now; I let go without thinking just as her tears stopped. About a hundred miles later the landscape went blurry and I had to stop again while Linda held me.

I knew that Linda was still thinking about the kid, and would for some time. Not me. To me, he had been generic protoplasm frozen in time; only if he had become ours would I have allowed him to turn into a real person with a past, present, future. Before we left the motel, Linda had told me that she couldn't go through another adoption ordeal. This kid had been our last chance at parenthood, and I couldn't bear for him to have space in my mental scrapbook if he wasn't going to show up in a real one.

Now that I wouldn't shape another person's life, I had to figure out how to make something more of my own. I had to change the shape of my existence so much that I could no longer see anyplace within it to fit in a child. Somehow I would come up with a plan that worked.

I would never know Ed the father, an image that had dominated my view of myself for nearly a decade, an image I'd sacrificed nearly everything else to become. I couldn't return to where I'd left off nine years before, yet I couldn't imagine what I'd move forward into.

As the snowcapped Rocky Mountains came into view, I thought of the last time I went skiing, twelve years before. It was a month before my thirtieth birthday, and I'd fallen and broken my hand at the end of the first run of the day. I'd begun my thirties with a cast on my hand, seeing the injury as a symbol of my loss of youth, of a future of continually diminishing returns. But a few days after my birthday, I had an epiphany of sorts. I told myself that, even though the length of my life was finite, its width wasn't. There was no limit to the things I could try to do, see, hear, learn, experience. I could expand my borders, make each day seem fuller and more rewarding, if I simply *chose* to.

The ability to make myself believe in something positive against all odds had become dangerous during the infertility, burying me in delusion and allowing my obsessive side to take over. But it had proved a great asset before that, bringing me to safe havens in the midst of other difficult situations over the years. Perhaps it would help me stake a claim in whatever future awaited me.

At least I wouldn't be doing it alone. Linda and I were finally on the same track again, released from the shaky alliance of the past decade. It would take time for the smoke to clear, but it would—I was sure of it. Then I'd be ready to take a clear look at the loyal and loving woman who had sacrificed so much through all this. Maybe I'd even get a better look at myself.

I kept driving.

# Chapter 13
# Someone Else's Child

We are on a flight home from Denver, and all the passengers except us look spunky and healthy, like Tovah Feldshuh with a tan. Ed's eyes are closed; he's probably doing a relaxation exercise. I'm going over and over in my mind what has happened to us in the last seventy-two hours. Once we're on the ground, everything will be firm and real. I need the ephemeral, suspension-of-disbelief state of flying through the air, the skin of the plane the only thing between me and the clouds, in order to convince myself of what has taken place.

We had flown out there like pilgrims, like nomads, wandering miles from home in search of treasure. I was excited by the adventure, but as it got closer I filled up with fear. When Ed and I settled in for the night in a hotel in Wyoming, headed for Nebraska and parenthood the next day, I felt little popping sensations up and down my chest. My hands were clammy and my heart was jumping. "Please God," I prayed as I lay in the strange bed in the dark, "make me able to love this little boy. For his sake. For Ed's sake."

We drove all the next morning until we were far from everything but the hospital where our two-day-old son lay. On the plane ride, we had narrowed the name choices down to two, but now we discarded them both and chose Alex instead. It sounded hard and durable, and had the traits of trustworthiness and wisdom I associated with Alex Rieger, Judd Hirsch's character from *Taxi.* We checked into a spartan room and called our lawyer. A meeting had been set up with Nellie and her lawyer in three hours, at 4:00. We expected to cool our heels until then, but our lawyer encouraged us to go to the hospital. Nellie had been discharged, but the newborn remained a patient. The nurses would be expecting us, and we could return to the hospital right after the meeting to pick Alex up and take him back to the motel with us. A few days' wait for interstate agreements and we'd be able to bring him home.

I had an idea that the nurses would be vaguely resentful of us. They probably envisioned us as wealthy, rude New Yorkers who always got everything they wanted. They could define us only by a name I had not yet firmly embraced: adoptive parents. We were surrounded by strangeness—the broad, undifferentiated landscape of this Midwestern state with its tumbleweeds rolling dryly across our path, its freight trains with uncountable numbers of cars, its ranches and cowboys—and by strangers: the girl who bore our child, the lawyers who would make him ours, these nurses who would hand him over.

A few minutes later we were driving along the town's wide, tree-lined main street, reminiscent of a 1950s downtown, and through a wrought-iron archway. The hospital was named for the shape of the butte in that part of the county and was so small that everything seemed to be on one floor. Once at the front desk, we were simply pointed toward Maternity. When we got there, we were identified even before we spoke—the clothes? the walk? the couple with the woman not in labor?—and approached by a gaggle of nurses. "It's a good thing you got here now," one of them said with a friendly smile. "That little boy is so beautiful, and he just loves to be cuddled. A few of us might just have taken him home ourselves." Their unexpected kindness and the bright, immaculate hospital suddenly made me feel that we were about to experience joy.

The nurses settled us in to a small, homey room, where they would bring our son in to us. I opened the blinds to let in the brilliant sun through the slats. When I turned back to face the room, the walls and floor were striped with sunlight, and a beaming nurse was wheeling him in on a hospital bassinet. "Which of you would like to hold him first?" she asked. "Ed?" I said, looking up at him with a smile, knowing how much he had craved this moment. The baby's eyes were closed and he had no eyebrows yet, but his head was covered with downy blond hair and he had a distinctive, squared-off nose and beautifully shaped lips.

They left the three of us alone, and Ed and I took turns holding our new son, incredulous at our good fortune and at how immediately lovable he was. He smelled of formula, powder, and new baby skin. We felt giddy, goofy, closer to laughter than tears. Over the next two hours, a young nurse taught us the practical part of being his parents. First we washed him down, starting with his eyes and ending with his tiny feet between our fingers as I raised him to clean his bottom. I took an alcoholed swab to his navel, where the umbilical cord stood black and rubbery. Ed put a fresh diaper on him and swathed him in hospital shirt and blankets. From time to time, with great effort, Alex lifted an eyelid to reveal a sea wave of deep blue. The nurse left again and we sat on the bed, transfixed, while the little boy fell asleep on my shoulder. He was ours! I was even fingerprinted as his mother, and a new birth certificate was made out listing Ed and me as the parents. How strange, I thought, that they would try to change the facts.

We lingered in the hospital. I asked to see the labor and delivery room, trying to fix in my mind every detail so that I could share it with Alex in years to come. Nellie had been "just great" during delivery, the nurse said. We found out that teenage pregnancy was rampant in the area; one hospital had seen a twelve-year-old mother. They invariably kept their babies. These nurses were delighted to see this young boy get off to a better start.

Finally, little Alex was wheeled back into the nursery. It was time for us to meet Nellie. The nurses filled my arms with diaper bags, bottles of formula, information about getting his picture taken. We were told to stop by the pediatrician's office next door before leaving. He turned out to be a crusty old transplanted Brooklynite, also glad to meet us. We asked each other a few questions and made an appointment to bring Alex in to him on Monday morning.

Ed and I walked out of the hospital grinning, giggling. These people, for no reward, were handing us our child, someone else's child who would now be ours. The sun felt hot for late March. There was a steady wind, the prairie breeze, but it only seemed to press the hot air closer to us.

* * *

I had wanted to return to our room to spruce up before meeting Nellie, but we had stayed at the hospital longer than expected; the visor mirror would have to do. I pulled out a few gray hairs—sixteen years old! What would we seem like to her? I was seven years older than her mother!—and balmed my prairie-dry lips. I was beginning to feel too hot under my woolen pullover. In the parking lot, Ed and I hugged each other and squeezed each other's hands, then walked across the street to the lawyer's office.

The receptionist told us to wait right there in the storefront lobby. A few minutes after we took our seats, in walked a young woman in shorts and a ponytail, accompanied by a red-haired, red-faced man in a black cowboy hat. "Nellie?" I asked reflexively, then gave her a sisterly embrace when she replied. She introduced us to her stepfather, who would not look us in the eye. I asked a stream of questions about how she felt, all the while trying to freeze in my mind her precious features: the pale skin, the fawn coloring, that same squared-off nose I would come to know as well as my own.

Finally the lawyer arrived and led us down the hall to a meeting room. Nellie had requested to speak to us alone, he said. Her stepfather offered to stay, but she was firm. I admired her. She knew this would be the only occasion ever for the person who bore Alex and the ones who were going to raise him to speak directly. Her lawyer and stepfather left and closed the door behind them.

There we sat, under the stark fluorescent lights, Ed and I on one side of a broad table and she on the other. We talked about the birth ("It wasn't so bad"), about Nellie's plans (she wanted to go to college), about the boy's father (a "cowboy" she did not have a real relationship with and whose identity she wanted kept secret). She and I chattered back and forth like neighbors. Ed sat quietly, a bit awed and overcome. But I was a machine of support and advice, talking so animatedly and optimistically that I didn't pick up the signals until I finally heard an unmistakable phrase or two: "if I had met you sooner," "if I hadn't seen him after the birth."

She needed more time before signing the form, she said. I didn't miss a beat, though my head was pounding and the lights felt like the harsh Nebraska sun outside, without even the mock relief of a breeze. I kept asking questions, offering help, advising without influencing. There we three sat for an hour—me all big-sisterish, Ed silent and cautious, the chatty schoolgirl holding all the cards.

"Whatever I decide," she said with genuine sympathy, "it's not because of you two. You guys are great. It has nothing to do with you."

It had nothing to do with us.

Somehow the meeting drew to a close and the lawyer came back into the room. Nellie left to meet her stepfather at a fast-food place to talk. All the blood drained from my face and my heart. I felt hollowed, hardened, had.

The lawyer stayed behind to talk. "Have you seen Dalton?" he asked us. Who? Was there yet another stranger we needed to see, someone who held unsigned forms for us, someone who would never know us but would determine whether or not this boy would become the most important thing in our lives? Then it dawned. Nellie had, of course, chosen her own name for the baby, and it didn't occur to this lawyer—not even a real adoption attorney, just someone faxed and phoned into readiness by a specialist hours away in Omaha, someone wearing a cheap, ill-fitting suit and having a head of hair like a Brillo pad—didn't occur to him that uttering that name would bring the fantasy we had spun crashing down around us, roaring in our ears, finally reducing itself to a little pool at our feet.

We hadn't even left our seats, but we were already back home, closing the door to the new nursery, putting the suitcase of baby clothes into the attic, telling friends and family one by one that things hadn't worked out.

We walked, dazed, back across the street to the rented car. The freebie baby samples were still in the backseat. My sweater still held Alex's clean, powdery scent and the heavy odor of bottled formula. I closed my eyes and breathed in the smells slowly. It was hot, mercilessly hot, Meursault-hot. Ed and I didn't speak until we got back to the motel room, then we didn't speak some more. I assumed the pose of some Victorian lady with the vapors. The pain in my head was intense and diffuse, and I lay on the bed with a cold compress, a tall bottle of Tylenol at my side.

Ed and I felt a grief so private it wasn't even each other's. He escaped into sleep, drained and saddened. I lay awake, thinking of the precious little boy, unclaimed by any mother or father, though he had two of each. His future lay in the fluctuating thoughts of a high school junior. Had it only been the night before that I feared I wouldn't love him? Was I being tested? "Please God," I prayed on this new night in this new motel room, "please let us have him." She just needed more time. We had held him! He had been ours! He could still be ours!

In the morning, Ed wisely decided that we should take a long drive rather than sit by the phone. We were each still keeping our sorrow to ourselves. I stepped into the shower and squatted to test the temperature of the water from the faucet. As soon as it started flowing, so did my tears, the noise of the running water hiding my sobs. After a few minutes I heard Ed come into the bathroom and make some jaunty comment to the shower curtain about our day trip. When I didn't answer after a second and third "Okay, hon?" he pulled back the curtain. I couldn't yet look at him or gasp enough air to breathe properly. He reached me then, wrapping his sturdy, familiar arms around my crouched figure. I could feel his desperation, but I needed him to be strong and so he was.

During the day it was easy to fool ourselves—singing "Rocky Raccoon," stopping for coffee, pretending to be tourists. We were hungry for distraction. But when it got dark and Ed drove us all the way back to that airless town, the stars shone menacingly and we grew silent. I closed my eyes in the dark car, but all I could see was that baby boy: the heart of his red lips, the flap of his earlobe, and the blue, blue eye that had struggled to see me.

I prayed hard to a God I wasn't sure was listening. It reminded me of the time I was about twelve and had asked for a sign. Before getting into bed one night I'd placed a handkerchief in the middle of the floor, asking God to prove to me that he existed by removing it while I slept. As soon as I woke in the morning, I glanced down to see that it had disappeared. I felt radiant, singled out. A few minutes later I found it on top of my dresser; my mother, I guessed, had seen it when she opened my door at her bedtime and picked it up. I was cynical for a moment, then I reconsidered. It *had* been taken off the floor, after all. That was the sign I had asked for.

Ed phoned the lawyer as soon as we got back to the room. His voice sounded far away and soft. When he hung up, he turned to me and said flatly that Nellie had decided to keep her boy. Her Dalton, I thought. Numb with hurt and the relinquishing of anticipated dread for real dread, we hardly reacted. I had been living on Tylenol and cold compresses, and I simply took some more of both and lay down on the bed. The only thing we wanted to do was get out. I called the airline and moved up our flight. Then I called my sister Barbara to let someone know what had happened—I couldn't bear the thought of my family still feeling excitement and anticipation. I heard my voice, fatigued but efficient, saying simply, "She changed her mind." It was April Fool's Day, I realized.

When shock and heavy disappointment fall, all we can do is concentrate on the business at hand. I told the young couple at the front office that we would be checking out first thing in the morning. I figured they wondered why we had asked for a crib when they could see we had no baby, so, with surprising composure, I told them our story. For an instant I thought they'd be more sympathetic to their compatriot than to us, but they were fiercely on our side. I suddenly felt defensive for Nellie.

Back in our room, Ed and I walked around and past each other getting ready for bed. He fell into a heavy, coma-like sleep while I cried steadily, quietly, for hours in bed next to him. The room still smelled of sweet baby things.

Around midnight I got up, dressed, and gathered the samples of baby products. I sat at the little desk in the room and wrote a long note to the nurses at the hospital, thanking them and leaving our phone number in case they heard of another girl looking for adoptive parents. I told them they needed to let Nellie know that the baby had a doctor's appointment Monday morning at 10:00. Then I got in the car and headed down the main street. It was Saturday night and there were knots of teenagers hanging around each other's cars. How many of these young girls, I thought, would end up in Nellie's situation? Maybe even because of something that would happen that very night, jammed in the backseat of some young boy's car or sprawled in an open field, being breathed and sweated on, not getting any erotic pleasure, just thankful for the closeness and the momentary care.

I drove through the wrought-iron archway and into the hospital parking lot. This was a small country hospital at midnight: the front door was locked. So, laden with this booty I had no rights to, I walked around to the back door, aching for recognition and closure. I was on a mission. As absurd as I must have looked walking through the dark with my arms filled with baby products, I felt businesslike. Two nurses with puzzled looks and crossed arms watched me slowly emerge from the blackness. There would be a different shift on duty. I explained my business and, to my surprise, began to weep. They led me into the hospital and sat me down on a bench. Then they walked off and spoke softly together. I was an after-hours embarrassment, someone to be whispered about in the hallway.

One of them came back and sat with me. Even in my state, I was aware that she was saying all the wrong things, things that could only make me feel worse. "You know, sometimes the maternal instinct can kick in very hard once the baby is born." And: "Well, at least he looks like a strong, healthy thing. He'll need it to make it in that family." Yeah, thanks, I thought. Now I'm not only the jilted mother, but I fear for the boy's well-being. He'd be sleeping in his bassinet, only a few rooms away. For a split second I thought of asking her if I could say good-bye to him, but I stopped myself. Finally. I was going to stop.

I would look Ed in the eye and tell him in a calm voice, slowly, intentionally: "I cannot go through this again. You have got to hear me: I cannot go through this again." He could leave if he had to. He could get the child he couldn't live without. But it wasn't going to be with my help anymore. If we couldn't have Alex, we were not going to adopt another baby together.

On the drive back to the motel, my head felt clear. My mind had new space to wander in. Something, I realized all at once, had been floating around the edges of my consciousness for days; it suddenly flooded to its center. My head had been pounding, my breasts looked different, my period was late.

Now I understand why my capacity for sorrow seemed doubled when we had to give Alex up: my body had in it two hearts to break.

It was ridiculous, it was impossible, but I knew it was true: I was pregnant. The next morning Ed and I fled that motel room with its cramped sadness and got back in our rented car to retrace our steps. Ahead of us we had a long day's drive to let go of Alex and Nellie and the nurses and the sun-drenched room where we'd held a promise for a few hours.

After we checked into a motel in Denver, I convinced my skeptical and distraught husband that we needed to pick up a pregnancy test. It was nothing but a stick. All you had to do was pee on it and wait three minutes. As Ed set the timer on his watch, I could already see the blue chemical reaction beginning to reveal itself. He'd need those three minutes, though, so I didn't say anything. And he'd need all that was left of the nine months. As for me, I was ready.

# Chapter 14
# Nine Years, Nine Months

Visibility through the windshield is poor, but I can see all the way to Pluto in this snowstorm, to the end of the universe. Both of my hands grip the steering wheel, in the ten-and-two position. I will follow every rule I learned in driver's ed twenty-five years ago. Steadiness is more important than speed right now, and finally I have my steadiness back. No tremors in the hands, no racing pulse, even though this is when men are supposed to have them—when they're driving their wives to the hospital to give birth to their first child.

The memory of my ride through the stark Nebraska landscape eight months ago can't hurt me now; it's been upgraded from tragedy to irony after one of my sperm somehow moored itself to one of Linda's eggs, without high-tech drugs or ray guns or spells conjured by sorcerers. How had it happened? No one would ever be able to explain.

I had feared Linda might be unraveling back in that Denver motel room when she said we needed to get a pregnancy test, less than twenty-four hours after our adoption fell through. When I saw with my own eyes the unmistakable blue line on the test stick, I thought her insanity was contagious. How could I possibly take that in? Linda had been pregnant all along: during the conversations with Nellie, during the afternoon we held that infant boy in our arms, during that agonizing drive through miles of nothingness when I thought my dream of parenthood was officially dead. I kept bouncing back and forth between disbelief and relief, suspicion and elation. Then finally there was no bouncing—just the rippling of Linda's belly as our unborn child went for its evening swim.

I look up at the sky and smile. We hadn't known it was snowing during the night. We'd been so busy monitoring the drumroll inside Linda that we never looked out the window. After coming outside to start the car, I launched a few four-letter protests at the sky but then started tittering. I knew that a mere storm couldn't hurt us. Nature was powerful, but it didn't stand a chance against a miracle.

While waiting at a stoplight, I follow the fall of a single snowflake onto my windshield. That is what the trauma of the last nine years has become: compressed into a tiny dot in my head. I know that this tiny dot will not melt, that it will have to be explored eventually and perhaps has the power to expand again. But for now, it can do nothing but serve as the period at the end of a very long sentence.

I ask Linda something in the car. She waves me off. The contractions are too strong for her to talk. There's so much to say, but it can wait.

Soon most of our talk will be gibberish aimed at a bassinet. We will forget how to talk to each other like adults, just as all new parents do for a while. Someday, though, we'll have the conversation we should have had years ago but put aside for reasons that sometimes made sense, often didn't. Someday we'll talk about all of it. But certainly not now.

I know that the joys of parenthood awaiting me will not erase the scars of the past nine years. I'm willing to confront those scars, to try to learn whatever lessons they can teach me about myself and my marriage. But not until our new baby is woven tightly into the fabric of my new life.

The snow is accumulating. Schools will be closed. My child's first day of life will be a snow day. I like this; it makes it seem like a holiday. As we take her outside for the first time, she'll think the whole world is this enchanting, clean place covered in fairy dust.

Every mile or so I see another car stuck in a snowbank on the side of the road. This will not happen to me. I am Moses crossing the Red Sea.

I'm turning onto the exit for the hospital. A plow is clearing the road up ahead. The snow is no longer snow, but confetti. God is staging a parade to honor our new child.

What I have longed for is about to emerge from its hiding place. It will be flesh and blood, tangible to all my senses, instead of a picture in my head that has been drawn, crossed out, redrawn, and erased over the last decade.

It will be Julia.

# Epilogue

"You were born in a snowstorm," I will tell Julia when she is old enough to understand. "It snowed so hard the day you were born, we didn't think we'd make it to the hospital on time." We were about nine years late, actually, but we made it in time to huff and push and wonder, as all parents have before us.

Did all the ovulation-enhancing, endometriosis-reducing, varicocele-shrinking techniques culminate in our ability to pull this off ourselves? Or would it have happened even if Ed and I had just met and fallen into bed for the first time the day she was conceived? Of all the unanswered medical questions in my mind, those were the most confounding.

But no thought was funnier to me than this: Julia was an accident. We hadn't even been trying to conceive for two years. I believe it was a hilarious fluke, although it didn't hurt that Ed and I made love like teenagers that spring, settled in a new house and free of the strictures of our fertility rituals.

Something opened in me that spring. Call it maternal instinct or biological imperative or just my cervix finally ready to let something through. I knew from the EPT moment in that hotel room that this would be our viable pregnancy. Poor Ed turned white with shock. I laughed uproariously. And laughed again at my postpartum visit when the obstetrician asked me what form of birth control we were now using. ("After ten years? You've got to be kidding!") And again whenever people ask us if we'd like to have another. ("At nine years per," I tell them, "I'll be pushing fifty by the next one, so I don't think so.")

And if we hadn't conceived? Ed tells me he'd seen the failed adoption as the end of the line, too, because I'd finally said, "Enough." We would have survived, together, the two of us. We would have found it in ourselves to reclaim what we needed, to pull our heads back in from the window and just enjoy the ride.

I'd been through a milder, though longer, blitz than the one my mother had lived through in London in the forties. Like her, I was grateful just to be out of the war zone, and, like her, I'd experienced the defining era of my life—the years around which every memory would fall "before" or "after."

I felt bad in a way that the pregnancy had come about without Dr. Gold's help. It took him several days to return my call leaving the news. When he did, we spoke briefly. I could feel the miles between us. He was happy for Ed and me, but there was something tamped down, weary, about his response. I asked him how I could possibly have gotten pregnant on my own, and he said, "Given enough time and enough luck, even serious problems can be overcome. I always hoped something like this would happen to you two." Now I often drive by the two-tone building where I was his patient, Julia chattering in her car seat. I can't pass it without remembering everything that went on in there, and in a strange way sometimes missing it. I'd been pregnant only nine months, but infertile for nine years. I would always identify more closely with the infertility.

Among the gifts Julia has given us—the perspective and the indispensability, the new capacities for love and new sense of ineptness—one I particularly treasure is an image I would never have had in my mind if I hadn't spent uncounted hours in a rocking chair with her. When I would emerge from my bed deep in the night to nurse her, I'd sense a connection with other mothers everywhere, past and present, as we watched the sun rise together, watched the snowflakes tumble, watched our cherished bundles take nourishment. It made me think of myself as an infant in my mother's arms, made me wonder how similar to Julia I looked and acted.

But more: I allowed myself to imagine my mother and my father as infants in their parents' arms. Before the hurt, the cruelties, the punishments and damage. They, too, had once been welcomed and cherished. They, too, started out new, when other possibilities beckoned. My mother, before she made the decisions she felt she had to live with, before life punished that sweet, meek woman for her sweetness and meekness. My father, before he grew to see life as something he had to fight his way through all alone. A simple thought: they had been infants once, in the distant 1920s. But a thought I would never have had if I'd never held my own child to me, a tiny woodland creature with creamy skin and dark, alert eyes.

And all the rest of it. The bone-crushing exhaustion. The fresh new skin to kiss and caress. The sheer *physicality* of the whole undertaking for someone with as still a center as mine. The moments when I wonder how Ed and I will cope with raising a child in our forties, and how I will wear the mantle of mother after the long and violent voyage to it. Watching Ed in the role he was born for, devoted, rewarded, finally free of the compulsion of the dream. Our marriage battered but intact—if not stronger in the places it was broken, at least mending.

I look at him, at that face I know so well, that face I will watch or imagine in my last moments, and see how almost ashen it sometimes looks, how his features are going fuzzy around the edges. The thin pleats around my own eyes, the gray hairs grown too numerous to pluck. We are heading into middle age together, losing the definitive lines our faces and hearts showed in our youth. Partnered as young lovers, now partnered in the love of a new child. Like all parents, making it up as we go along, creating a way to connect with this giggling, gorgeous, curly-headed, defiant child.

I don't let myself worry yet about whether Julia will be able to have her own babies one day. I can hardly remember the fainting spells during the pregnancy, the dire first weeks with a newborn, the shocking loss of time and the overpowering responsibility. What I remember is this: flying home late one evening from a visit with Ed's family in Arizona with my one-year-old sound asleep in my lap. Dear God, I say to myself, when it is time for you to take me, let it feel like this: suspended in space, enfolded in love, no longer where I've been but not yet where I'm going, the lovely, breathing weight of my sleeping child pressing against me. I will be ready to go then. Please take me then.

# Acknowledgments

A lot of people helped us through the living and the writing of this story. I'd like to extend deep gratitude to Elaine Edelman, whose wonderful workshops at The Writer's Voice gave me the permission and the tools I needed to begin writing. To my treasured friends and colleagues at Basic Books, who helped us shape the proposal and find an agent: Jo Ann Miller, Susan Rabiner, Gail Winston, Paul Golob, and especially Juliana Nocker Ferry, whose exuberance makes all things seem possible and who was a major factor in getting us off our butts after years of thinking about doing a book. To Roberto de Vicq de Cumptich for his graciousness and friendship. To Phoebe Hoss, who showed me what it means to be an editor and who got me a job as her replacement at Basic, where I honed my editing and writing skills on other people's books. To Mike Mueller, who gave me a blank journal for Christmas 1993 in which I wrote what eventually became the first chapter of this book. And who, in perfect symmetry, arranged in 1998 for me to have a luxurious week alone in an apartment on Sixteenth Street to finish up my half. Much thanks to Shaill Jhaveri for his incredible generosity to a stranger.

To my sisters, Janet Carbone and Barbara Botta, for their invaluable support and honesty, and my parents, Violet and Nicholas Carbone, who have always done right by me. To Ivy Miller, whose cherished friendship, keen perspective, and sophisticated editorial eye are deeply appreciated. To Kathleen Ryan LiCastri, who always gave me a friend's honest reaction and a patient ear during the struggle. To Mary and David Ziller, for a golden friendship and a couple of stories repeated here. To our fertility doctor, referred to in these pages as David Gold: thank you for everything, especially your devoted medical care and your delightful personality. And for answering all my questions during the treatment and the book writing. You still have my sacred trust. (I hope I still have yours.)

To Lauren Schultz, my hilarious and bighearted friend who grew up with me and whose useful memory helped me describe that world. To the fabulous women of SGP, who kept me laughing and made sure I had other things to be frantic about during the months most of these chapters were written: Robin Dellabough, Lisa DiMona, Sarah Silbert, Karen Watts, and especially Ann Weinerman, a dear new friend I am old enough to be the mother of, if only I hadn't been infertile.

We were extremely fortunate to have found a generous and enthusiastic agent in Arielle Eckstut at James Levine Communications. (And thanks to Jim Levine, who offered to represent us the same day he received our proposal.) And to have the astute editorial guidance and unflagging enthusiasm of two editors at the Atlantic Monthly Press, Anton Mueller and Elisabeth Schmitz. We'd also like to thank Morgan Entrekin, Judy Hottensen, Charles Woods, and Lissa Smith for their accessibility and expertise.

My final and biggest thanks go to my husband. I wouldn't want to go through the infertility *or* the co-authoring again (I think the latter was the more stressful), but thanks for making sure we survived both. They say that husbands and wives who live together for a long time begin to resemble each other. I hope to grow to resemble your sweet forbearance, your resilience, and the selfless principles on which your life is built. My heart is yours. (My uterus I think I'll keep to myself at this point.)

To anyone who lived through part of this with me and has a different memory of it, I apologize. This is what it looked like from where I was standing.

To all the couples in fertility treatment, straining to grasp the brass ring and not yet past their agonies, my heart goes out. May you reach resolution quickly.

And to Julia, who was underfoot and overhead during the writing of this book. This was all for you, dove.

—L. C.

I want to give special thanks to Elaine Edelman for her expertise as a writing instructor and for showing me how to access the closely guarded secrets of my inner self. I also want to thank Gay French-Ottaviani, whose innovative acting classes taught me how to draw on my deepest emotions when expressing myself. Our dear friend Ivy Miller helped me close the gap between the real me and the me portrayed in the book, with her incisive comments on my early drafts. Stefan Kanfer also provided invaluable advice and enthusiastic support—while also keeping my reflexes sharp as a formidable Ping-Pong opponent.

We were lucky to benefit from the keen insights of two immensely talented editors at the Atlantic Monthly Press, Anton Mueller and Elisabeth Schmitz. Our wonderful agent, Arielle Eckstut, provided valuable guidance and enthusiasm through the entire writing process.

For their continuing empathy and understanding during our ordeal, I'm forever thankful to my parents, Helen and David Decker, and my sister, Chris Cipolaro, and her family. My good friends Mike Podwill and Meg and Dennis Puccio were also bastions of support. To "Dr. Gold" I extend my thanks for his medical skill, warmth, and humor in helping us navigate the infertility maze.

Most of all, I want to express my undying gratitude and love to my wife and co-author. She is the key to my greatest happiness. My chapters are twice as effective as they would have been, thanks to her formidable skills as a reader and editor.

Finally, I want to thank the person who gave us the happy ending to our saga: our precious sweetie, Julia. She was well worth the wait.

—E. D.